D0398502

THE GENETICS OF HEALTH

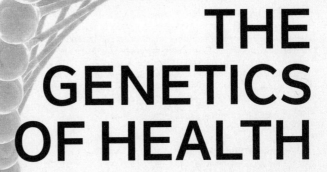

THE
GENETICS
OF HEALTH

Understand Your Genes for Better Health

SHARAD P. PAUL, MD

ATRIA BOOKS
New York London Toronto Sydney New Delhi

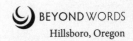
Hillsboro, Oregon

ATRIA BOOKS

An Imprint of Simon & Schuster, Inc.
1230 Avenue of the Americas
New York, NY 10020

BEYOND WORDS

20827 N.W. Cornell Road, Suite 500
Hillsboro, Oregon 97124-9808
503-531-8700 / 503-531-8773 fax
www.beyondword.com

This publication contains the opinions and ideas of its author. It is intended to provide helpful and informative material on the subjects addressed in the publication. It is sold with the understanding that the author and publisher are not engaged in rendering medical, health, or any other kind of personal professional services in the book. The reader should consult his or her medical, health, or other competent professional before adopting any of the suggestions in this book or drawing inferences from it. The author and publisher specifically disclaim all responsibility for any liability, loss, or risk, personal or otherwise, which is incurred as a consequence, directly or indirectly, of the use and application of any of the contents of this book.

Managing editor: Lindsay S. Easterbrooks-Brown
Editors: Ali McCart, Nevin Mays
Copyeditors: Gretchen Stelter, Emmalisa Sparrow Wood
Proofreader: Madison Schultz
Cover design: Devon Smith
Composition: William H. Brunson Typography Services

First Atria Books/Beyond Words hardcover edition April 2017

For more information about special discounts for bulk purchases, please contact Simon & Schuster Special Sales at 1-866-506-1949 or business@simonandschuster.com.

The Simon & Schuster Speakers Bureau can bring authors to your live event. For more information or to book an event, contact the Simon & Schuster Speakers Bureau at 1-866-248-3049 or visit our website at www.simonspeakers.com.

Manufactured in the United States of America

10 9 8 7 6 5 4 3 2 1

Library of Congress Cataloging-in-Publication Data

Names: Paul, Sharad P., author.
Title: The genetics of health : understand your genes for better health /
   Sharad P. Paul.
Description: New York : Atria ; Hillsboro, Oregon : Beyond Words, [2017] |
   Includes bibliographical references.
Identifiers: LCCN 2016050053 (print) | LCCN 2016051602 (ebook) |
   ISBN 9781501155413 (hardback) | ISBN 9781501155420 (paperback) |
   ISBN 97815011555437 (eBook)
Subjects: LCSH: Human genetics. | Alternative medicine. | Health. | BISAC:
   HEALTH & FITNESS / Healthy Living. | HEALTH & FITNESS / Alternative
   Therapies. | HEALTH & FITNESS / Health Care Issues.
Classification: LCC QH431 .P358 2017 (print) | LCC QH431 (ebook) | DDC
   616/.042—dc23
LC record available at https://lccn.loc.gov/2016050053

The corporate mission of Beyond Words Publishing, Inc.: *Inspire to Integrity*

For Natasha

CONTENTS

Introduction

A SCIENTIFIC WALKABOUT FOR WELLNESS

If this were so; if the desert were "home"; if our instincts were
forged in the desert; to survive the rigours of the desert—
then it is easier to understand why greener pastures pall on us;
why possessions exhaust us, and why Pascal's imaginary man
found his comfortable lodgings a prison.

—Bruce Chatwin

The development of our species is still a veritable work-in-progress. For humans living in the present, and indeed for any creature, our present is like a photograph, and our species seems eternal. This dangerous illusion keeps our focus away from the invisible photographer called time, which chronicles the story of our evolution in black and white, so it can be reproduced as a testament to our biological era at a later date.

We humans are essentially vain creatures who have developed a penchant for self-imagery. But is this evolutionary self-photograph unintentionally symbolic? Man is placed at the top of the image, with many creatures underneath. Yet no one seems to be moving, which is reasonable since this is a photograph.

Studying evolutionary biology is merely poring over an old selfie, where background matters less and the environment ends up a mere prop for the individual. Extinction always seems to happen to other animals; that's why our ancestors and other extant and extinct species matter. They need to be remembered—because lessons we learn, or don't heed, can be the doing or undoing of our species.

One of my many academic roles is at the School of Medicine, University of Queensland, Australia. In Australia, "going walkabout" refers to a rite of passage that the Aboriginal people undertake—a time of solitude spent searching for "songlines" of their ancestors—the idea being to imitate the past and return with renewed energy to face the future.

In traditional Australian Aboriginal thinking, there exists a "creation era" and "creation ancestors"—if you think about it, these concepts pretty much sum up both the early evolution of life and the later migration of populations around the world. In the past, due to visceral bias rather than scientific discomfort among some researchers, people searched for alternative explanations of our ancestral origins. Surely, the Europeans couldn't have originated in *black* Africa—even though research shows that Homo erectus, the first upright human beings, made their appearance about 1.9 million years ago, and they were followed by Homo neanderthalensis (Neanderthals), and finally by Homo sapiens (modern humans), our common race.

Vincent van Gogh once said, "Looking at stars always makes me dream, as simply as I dream over the black dots representing towns and villages on a map." He mused that while we could take a train to travel between towns, we had to take death to reach a star. But life is to be lived, cherished, and enjoyed, not something we merely exist through. Birth and death are natural inevitabilities—it is the in-between that we have control over. But there is no map that can illustrate the fickleness of human behavior. That's why songlines matter; our history makes us more than we make history.

One of the best known songlines in Australia is the Dreaming Story of Seven Sisters—this saga is set in the constellation Taurus and is the story of "seven star sisters" that make up the cluster we now call Pleiades.[1] In different tribes and, more recently, in different art galleries across Australia, the interpretation of this story varies slightly, but the theme is the same—seven sisters are running away from a Jampijinpa man, a stalker who wants to take one of these sisters as his wife. The sisters flee across the continent, and in the end, they climb up a steep mountain, launch themselves into the sky, and become stars; every night these seven sisters jump into the night sky, pursued by the Jampijinpa man, who follows them.

Studying this particular Aboriginal songline interested me, especially the part about seven women becoming stars, because there is a parallel seven sisters European songline in evolutionary biology— the story of mitochondrial DNA (mtDNA) that can be traced back to seven women.

Mitochondria are the powerhouses of our cells, and we know that they probably once existed as independent organisms that somehow learned to generate energy and, therefore, got gobbled up by greedy, single-celled creatures in the early parts of the story of life. While males also have mitochondrial DNA, it does not get passed on; therefore, each of us inherits this mtDNA from our mother, who in turn inherited her mtDNA from her mother, and so on. Therefore, all women can be traced back to one woman, the proverbial Eve.

However, once about every thousand generations, point mutations occur in this mtDNA, and what we've ended up with is that all modern populations of European origin can be classified into seven different genetic populations based on their mitochondrial heredity. In his book *Seven Daughters of Eve*, Brian Sykes points out that while each of these "clan mothers" lived several thousand years apart, they all shared a common ancestor: the mitochondrial Eve.[2] So there are, in fact, seven mitochondrial sisters; life imitates art after all.

If most of the stars and genes have been mapped, where does that leave us? Do we simply succumb to our astrological or genetic fate? The truth is, even people who believe in fate or destiny have to look both ways while crossing the road. Environment matters a great deal. Just as our genes shape what we do to our surroundings, our environment, in turn, modifies our genes. Genetics and evolutionary biology are songlines of what makes us human and healthy.

There's a fundamental difference between medicine and health. Modern Western medicine works on an illness model—you have a disorder that gets cured, either by taking a chemical or by undergoing a procedure. But we know that, in some cases, even placebos can work if we believe we are taking the real thing, especially for symptom control. We often underestimate the power of our minds, the impact of the stress response, or how eating or drinking too much affects our overall health—we all have our own Jampijinpa men pursuing us across the sky.

Health demands some personal discipline. We cannot place complete faith in the medical industry at the expense of our own individual health. We won't find good health in medicines, be they derived synthetically or naturally. Drugs are meant for curing certain conditions or alleviating symptoms, not as sustenance. Even in the wellness industry, there are people pushing unscientific products. So it is our responsibility to understand our wellness—and to do this, we need to look back at our collective pasts, our individual genetic differences, and understand the thin line between mind and body fitness. Sometimes we have to look back before we can move forward.

Last year, I was reading *Walkabout*, an Australian classic, to some schoolchildren, which contains the below passage:

There was a time to be weaned, a time to be carried in arms;
a time to walk with the tribe, a time to walk alone; a time for
the proving of manhood, a time for the taking of gins . . . these
things were done in order.[3]

I realized that it was time for me to go on my own walkabout for wellness. I took my time and wandered into the forests of academia, trying to see the forest for the trees. I became more and more curious about the evolutionary biology of our pasts, and my perspective changed—it was not just about where our ancestors hunted or what they ate, but also how these things shaped our genes. This book is that songline, the story of our one human race having conversations with our individual and familial pasts that, in turn, end up being blueprints for our personal and personalized health. I call this the (R_X)Evolutionary Road that leads to good health.

This book is structured so each chapter takes a look at a specific set of genes and its role in our bodies—movement, stress response, weight, pigment, and digestion—explores their evolution, and provides practical advice for pursuing health in today's world. In my twenty-eight years as a medical doctor, I have never lost a working day due to illness. In the beginning, I didn't think this was unusual—but everyone else seemed to think so, especially given my busy schedule, stressful surgical work, and amount of international travel. It does not mean injury or illness cannot fell me tomorrow. But being healthy in body and mind means that you can live life to the fullest. A magazine called *Hum* once featured me on their cover under the headline "Sharad Paul: Living Life to the Full." I was surprised when I read that. I simply do things I am passionate about, and that gives me energy. I agree with Oprah Winfrey when she says, "Passion is energy."[4]

With this book, my mission is to learn and teach, to become both the message and messenger. This book has many ideas, resources, and suggestions for you. But fundamentally this is *about* you—your past and how that can lead you forward to better health: how to eat for your gene type, what exercises to do, how to handle stress. It will then be your turn to go on your own wellness walkabout, as being healthy is not merely living a medicine-free life; health is life itself.

As someone who has written both fiction and nonfiction, I am often asked about the process of writing. In each book, an author has a favorite line. In my latest novel, *The Kite Flyers* (Harper Collins, 2014), there is this passage: "Old friendships are a tunnel into our past. No one should ask questions in a tunnel. Tunnels echo too much." In the course of these wanderings for wellness, I came across many tunnels and realized I had to ask many questions, even if the answers surprised my scientific mind. After all, biology has no bigotry—it welcomes both doubters and believers into its fold. As a physician and scientist, I had to listen carefully and make sure I was transcribing these evolutionary echoes. Those words are the ones I have repeated here, about food and fitness, hunger and health, mind and matter—things essential for the enjoyment of life's goodness, a desire that gnaws in us all.

1

THE ME AND WE GENES: MAKING EVOLUTION PERSONAL

The individual has always had to struggle to keep from being overwhelmed by the tribe. If you try it, you will be lonely often, and sometimes frightened. But no price is too high to pay for the privilege of owning yourself.

—Friedrich Nietzsche

As Nietzsche put it, there exists an evolutionary battle between the species and the individual. But there is also a similar yet smaller battle that happens inside our cells daily. Genes cling on to our chromosomes, which encode our heredity—they may hold some secrets, but they fundamentally lack deceit. To even think genes can be evil is to consider them a form of human expression, and they are not. Genes do what genes do. Their protein machinations outline the story of your life—context, character, and conflict resolution—but allow you to be the writer and forge your own plot or destiny. But just as creatures do, genes exist in different forms due to mutations (deviant versions of genetic codes), polymorphism (different forms of a gene that arise by mutation and are able to take on different embodiments), or alleles (different forms or twins of a gene that control specific traits, such as eye or hair color).

Therefore, certain genes emerge for the good of the species, while others are variably expressed in individuals. Humans used to be born free and lived collective communal lives—in neighborhoods that had neither national boundaries nor measurements of individual achievement. Then, our societies became more narrow, a fundamentally different direction for both man and gene. The strange thing about animal life is that, if you put any other animal in a pen, they go crazy. So in some ways, genes evolved for free populations. Humans voluntarily enclose ourselves—within fences and locked homes. Here's the other thing—all other animals try and control their populations to preserve the environment for their long-term benefit. Creatures like crocodiles can even determine the sex of their offspring by controlling incubation temperatures (i.e., burying eggs at different depths). In nature, the default choice for babies is female; males are largely superfluous beings. Humans are the only species in which males seem to dominate, and sadly, in many Asian countries, female infants or fetuses are still being killed.

We have now ended up in a globalized, male-dominated world where our genes, unsure of our existential purpose, are possibly trying to make us someone else. This age of travel and the internet means we have the ability to choose mates from different geographical environments, and no matter who we choose as a mate, our genes and those of our offspring are exposed to varying diets and environmental influences, which, in turn, affects those genes. While every human is an unprecedented individual, our ability to modify the genetic cards nature has dealt us by simply modifying our diets allows us to escape the heredity of ill health. Even brutal genes don't result in brutal humans. Evolution may involve violence, and even the killing off of certain species, but no one is held captive by their genes. Believers in both God and genes think of the creation process as someone mold-ing life with bare hands. But evolution is filled with flux and fantasy. It may be better to visualize it as artwork, and the real beauty of this creation lies in the eyes of a beholder—or biologist.

Within the sphere of medicine, we know that some things that are good for the species may not necessarily work for an individual. For example, breastfeeding is the best method of reducing fertility across a population, because hormonal changes during lactation lower a woman's reproductive capability; however, for an individual, that isn't a reliable or foolproof method of contraception. Biology has no favoritism; humans do. And beyond that, our genetic makeup means that some individuals respond differently to medications, even sham drugs.

Evolution and the "Me" Gene

A few years ago, I engaged a plumber to put a new toilet in our home. He had cut out a hole in the wall for drainage pipes, and one night, he forgot to plug the hole. Because we lived close to the sea, with a creek running through our property and plenty of bushland, a rat decided to visit our new room. This was before we had Zack, our Swedish Vallhund dog, a breed used for ratting in Sweden. On the discovery of rat droppings and other signs of an unwelcome guest, and concerned that this rat might have brought its family of gnawers in search of a warmer home, I called a pest-control guy. He placed some rat bait around the house and asked me if we had a dog.

"No," I said. "What difference would that make?"

"If a dog gets at the bait, then I'd have some vitamin K handy."

That's what we give patients who overdose on warfarin, I thought.

After the pest disappeared, I opened one of the containers the man had set around the house to find a bunch of warfarin pills, not even sweetened or anything like that. Rats aren't fussy. Obviously, the idea is to overdose a rat on warfarin and make it bleed to death.

Warfarin is one of the most common blood-thinning drugs used worldwide. Yes, men and women are prescribed this rat poison to thin their blood and prevent blood clots. When we screen patients prior to surgery at my skin cancer surgical practice, I am astounded how many older folk are on this rat poison, which is mostly prescribed to prevent blood clots caused by irregular heartbeats. The general population on warfarin grew dramatically from 1993 to 2008, from 0.63 percent to 2.28 percent, and since skin cancer mostly affects the elderly, I encounter a decent amount of patients on that drug.[1]

In ancient times, physicians used leeches to thin blood. About a century ago, Jay McLean, a medical student at Johns Hopkins, was credited with discovering heparin, which he extracted from animal liver. Then, coumarin was discovered. This chemical is found naturally in sweet clover that is often used as animal feeds. However, when afflicted with a fungus, coumarin becomes dicoumarol, a naturally occurring anticoagulant that depletes vitamin K and thereby induces bleeding; cows had been noted to die of internal bleeding after eating sweet clover contaminated by fungus. This finding led to synthetically produced warfarin—a drug that was discovered at the University of Wisconsin, hence the name: WARF is the acronym for the Wisconsin Alumni Research Foundation, and the ending -arin was because it was essentially a derivative of coumarin.

One of the issues with taking blood-thinning medications to prevent embolism (a blockage in the blood vessel) is that patients vary widely in their responses to drug therapy and often end up with serious and unpredictable complications. I was interested in looking at the blood thinners clopidogrel (commonly used in coronary disease to prevent clots after stents or surgery) and warfarin because such drugs have a "narrow therapeutic index"—medical jargon for a drug that has a small margin of error between toxic and therapeutic (treatment) doses and therefore needs to be closely monitored. Further, because of the variability of responses in patients, anticoagulants are the best medications to implement personalized drug treatment—in other words, medication dosing for your gene type.

Variance in warfarin toxicity can be explained by inheritable differences in the gene CYP2C9, which is linked to the cytochrome P450 superfamily of enzymes. Likewise, studies now show that people with an allelic variant—meaning those with different traits or characteristics on a particular chromosome, in this case, the loss-of-function variant of the CYP2C19 (CYP2C19*2) gene, another member of the cytochrome P450 family—had reduced platelet inhibition activity with clopidogrel and, therefore, higher rates of cardiac events, particularly thrombosis (when a blood clot fully blocks a vessel).

Now that genetic testing is easily available, I believe that more and more drug prescriptions will be tailored to your gene type in the future. As early as 2007, the FDA recommended genetic testing in patients to predict response to warfarin. Such personalized dosing will be used for more drugs as dosage based on individual genetic variations becomes more commonplace in mainstream medicine.

We often refer to millennials as the "Me" generation—more self-obsessed, less self-aware. Perhaps genes simply have to follow suit, to mimic the hosts, delivering arbitrary cellular commands to today's generation, a generation of people who are no longer in unions or united, but are instead reliant on technology that somehow hacks populations together. In the last fifty thousand years, as people migrated and adopted different diets, these habits caused the expression of new genes in certain populations. In some cases, society became the gene maker, rather than the individual, leading to collective genetic variations in certain populations.

Evolution and the DD Effect

In the past fifty thousand years, we have entered a phase of especially rapid evolution. Compared to other primates, human gene regulation has changed very quickly due to what I have termed "the DD effect," that is, due to demographics and diaspora.

On one hand, the massive population expansion has produced enough genetic mutants that natural selection has become outpaced; on the other, people have migrated from their origins, and diets and behaviors have largely become enveloped by sameness. With globalization, one can now find pizza or pad thai or paella anywhere in the world. But that's not how we evolved. Our genes are microscopic robotic coding machines that prepare us for the future that has been foretold, which is not necessarily how things turn out.

We earlier discussed how drug responses vary between individuals due to their gene types. As humans roamed the earth, they developed skin color changes (more about this later) and adopted nationhood that ultimately imposed restrictions on movement. With this also came more inbreeding. Therefore, certain population groups also have certain susceptibility when it comes to drugs.

We discussed blood-thinning medications earlier and the CYP2C19*2 gene variant. CYP2C19 is one of the principal enzymes involved in deactivating the blood thinner clopidogrel by the liver. The abnormal variants are carried in only 2 percent of the the Caucasian populations; African Amercans are twice as likely to carry this gene variant at 4 percent, but this is dwarfed by the 14 percent of Chinese people who are affected.

The reason evolutionary biology is so important to understanding various diseases is that, as evolution has progressed, it has left behind a trail of conserved ancient genes—and while we may change our lifestyles and environments, we cannot escape our pasts. Many of our genes were shaped by the diets and lifestyles of our ancestors. Essentially, genes involved in basic biochemical and anatomical alterations have largely remained constant over seventy thousand years, even if they may express themselves differently—and for a student of genetics or evolutionary biology, this fact provides both balance and a reason to investigate our past.

The thing about genes is, as the noted scientist Richard Dawkins says, they are inherently selfish—the survival of the fittest for a gene is basically everything to ensure *its* survival, and not the sustainability of the host.[2] There are millions of genes, often named as abbreviations of the functions of the proteins they encode. Inside each cell, genes hold memories, lying dormant and waiting to crackle to life, of populations past. This means behavior is often predetermined—my dog still circles his bed and ruffles the sheets vigorously as if he is trampling vegetation or creating a snow cave as his ancestors did. At the same time, just as genes shape our behavior, our behavior shapes our genes—the beauty of scientific nature or nurture has an underlying genetic bias. Our present environment, both internal and external, gives us an opportunity to fine-tune our genes, whether it's for dairy tolerance or the fight-or-flight instinct. But without scientific knowledge of our past, we end up a tree without strong roots.

At the Dalkey Book Festival in Dublin, I met John Banville, the celebrated Irish writer and author of *The Sea*. In his book, there is a line that stands out for me: "The past beats inside me like a second heart." Let's be true to our hearts.

Selfish Genes, Helpful Humans

Nothing much happens in the gene world except for the manufacture of proteins and the biochemical changes that result. Everything is on a minuscule scale inside a cell, but it is the finest theater. In this theater, there are few practicable entrances but many exits. If you work hard enough, everything is escapable, even genealogy or terrifying Jampijinpa men.

In Richard Dawkins's book *The Extended Phenotype*, he argues that as far as genes are concerned, they only control the manufacture of proteins. The effect of a gene is then also determined by the behavior of the organism. In some ways, that makes perfect sense—you may have genes that indicate your risk for a particular disease, but your behavior and lifestyle can affect how successful this gene activation becomes.

As Dawkins explains: "An animal's behavior tends to maximize the survival of the genes 'for' that behavior."[3] Dawkins also speaks of "the selfish gene":

> Let us try to teach generosity and altruism, because we are born selfish. Let us understand what our own selfish genes are up to, because we may then at least have the chance to upset their designs, something that no other species has ever aspired to do.[4]

Basically, genes are in the business of making proteins—nothing more, nothing less. As far as genes are concerned, any improvement or detriment to your health is purely luck. But if genes are fundamentally selfish, does it make man basically ungenerous? The short answer is no.

In 2004, there was the massive tsunami in Thailand—a great wave that left a trail of destruction in fourteen countries and killed over two hundred thousand people. A Czech supermodel, Petra Nemcová, and her fiancé, Simon Atlee, a photographer, were on vacation in Thailand when the tsunami struck. All Petra remembers hearing was Simon screaming, "Petra, Petra." It was the last time she saw her boyfriend. Petra was left with broken bones, a smashed pelvis, and blood collections around her kidneys. People expected her to be paralyzed, but she recovered with time.

She returned to Thailand to see how she could help rebuild the lives of the children who were impacted by the natural disaster, knowing that after the emergency response was completed, they would soon be forgotten. It's similar to when a doctor discharges a patient from the hospital, and the patient's needs are forgotten. But what made Petra go back? People would assume that supermodels often function in a rarified air of diamond-crusted celebrity—models are supposed to be haughty and arrogant, are they not? But Petra's generosity has changed the lives of thousands of people. She used her fame to raise awareness, funds, and bring much-needed help.

Dacher Keltner is the founding director of the Greater Good Science Center and a professor of psychology at the University of California, Berkeley. Keltner studies generosity and genetics, and feels that because of our very vulnerable offspring, the fundamental task for human survival and gene replication may actually be to take care of others. In his book *Born to Be Good: The Science of a Meaningful Life*,[5] Keltner points out that Darwin mentions benevolence ninety-nine times in *The Descent of Man*, including this pivotal quote:

> For firstly, the social instincts lead an animal to take pleasure in the society of his fellows, to feel a certain amount of sympathy with them, and to perform various services for them . . . Such actions as the above appear to be the simple result of the greater strength of the social or maternal instincts than that of any other instinct or motive; for they are performed too instantaneously for reflection or for pleasure or even misery might be felt.[6]

It seems obvious that Darwin felt that our tendencies toward sympathy are both instinctual and evolved—and actually stronger than our instincts of self-preservation. That's what made Petra Nemcová go back to Thailand even before the disaster had fully abated.

Scientific research increasingly shows that the reason Homo sapiens conquered our planet was because of our ability to nurture people other than ourselves. And as with the genes for many other attributes, altruism may also have a genetic basis.

Professor Jordan Grafman at the National Institutes of Health led one of two studies in the mid-2000s that examined where in the brain the impulse to give originates, thereby shedding light on why it feels so good to help others.[7] Both studies asked people to make donations to charities and looked at the resulting brain activity using functional magnetic resonance imaging (fMRI), which creates images of the brain's activity by detecting physical changes, such as blood flow, resulting from the activity of neurons.

When the volunteers placed the interests of others before their own, the generosity activated a primitive part of the brain that usually lights up in response to food or sex—the prefrontal cortex. Donating made the brain's two reward systems work together: the midbrain ventral tegmental area (VTA), which is stimulated by food, sex, drugs, and money, and the subgenual area, which is stimulated when humans see babies and their romantic partners. These traits are for our own good; not only does this mean we help others, but there is also generally lower health risk in being addicted to generosity in comparison to alcohol or sex—in my years as a physician, no one has been admitted to the hospital for suffering from acute generosity!

Darwin's theory of evolution is all about population fitness, rather than physical fitness. Fitness of a population refers to the ability of a population to propagate its species—the ability to survive to reproductive age, find a mate, and produce offspring. As Darwin himself noted, generosity confers great advantage to a population's fitness.

The Paradox of Generosity is a book by sociologists Christian Smith and Hilary Davidson, who recently presented their Science of Generosity Initiative at Notre Dame University.[8] These researchers surveyed two thousand individuals over a five-year period. They interviewed and tracked the spending habits and lifestyles of forty families from different classes and races in twelve states. People who described themselves as "very happy" volunteered an average of 5.8 hours per month. Those who were "unhappy" only spent 0.6 hours helping others. And nearly half the people who were more giving were in excellent health (48 percent), as opposed to only one-third of the "ungenerous" (31 percent). In other words, there is a reason that giving and generosity need to be present for human survival, and our genes are obliging facilitators. We also now know that people who have certain variants of a gene called AVPR1a gave, on average, nearly 50 percent more money than those who do not have it. But due to the implications for our individual well-being, the solution to parsimony is not destiny but openhandedness because, as we've just discussed, miserliness only leads to misery.

Genetic Individualism

The study of our genes and those of our ancestors helps us see not just how our species has evolved over millennia, but also how our individual genetic makeups are unique and how they affect our lives. Genetic tests for many dietary and physical markers are now available, and I routinely arrange such tests for my clients, if they are interested. There is no doubt that this will become more commonplace and, in my view, preferable, as they can help us understand the importance of balanced and varied diets. Personalized healthcare based on our own individual genetic blueprint is already on the horizon—not only for prevention of diseases like diabetes and high blood pressure, but even individualized cancer therapy. The latter is already becoming common in the field of oncology, with many cancer treatments based on genetic markers.

Is there a gene for occupational predisposition? Some people consider the medical profession a calling; others, a business. Whatever it is, I was doomed—I often joke that this vocation was imprinted in my family's genes. My parents, grandparents on my mother's side, uncles, and aunts were doctors—surgeons, physicians, dermatologists, ophthalmologists, and psychiatrists. My pioneering grandmother studied medicine at a time when women completed the same course as men, but only men were allowed to be called doctors; women like my grandmother were euphemistically called "licensed medical practitioners."

When my grandmother studied medicine, there were no medications for high blood pressure treatment. Until the 1900s, arterial blood pressure was not even measured clinically. When my grandmother developed high blood pressure, she was aware of the seriousness of her condition, especially the untreatable complications.

My grandmother had had a career as a district medical practitioner in British India. Times weren't easy—she was constantly moved to different places, and it didn't help that she was not afraid to expose corruption when people employed by the health service were stealing and reselling medications. This may have caused her stress that contributed to her illness, but she shone a light for many others to follow, not just in my family. After all, we earn a living by what we get, but it is what we give that matters in the end.

Actually, my grandmother's death could possibly have been prevented but for a kind of medical nihilism. Until the 1960s, many prominent doctors believed that arterial disease was the cause of hypertension, rather than the result, and therefore did not treat the disease, scoffing that they'd be practicing "treatment of the manometer rather than of the patient."[9] Change takes time in guilds such as medicine, and to this day, preventable tragedies sometimes occur.

The relationship between high blood pressure and salt in the diet was discovered in 1904 in Paris by two medical students, Ambard and Beaujard, who originally thought it was the chloride in salt that was the problem, not the sodium. This led to the development of diuretics as test medications for high blood pressure in the 1940s. My grandmother had malignant hypertension (dangerously high blood pressure that resulted in severe organ damage). She could have been saved by such drugs had the medical profession understood the connection earlier and begun treating high blood pressure. In 1947, doctors began to attempt to treat malignant hypertension with the use of the World War II antimalarial agent pentaquine. Later, other more effective drugs were developed. But by the time they came around to southern India or became part of routine medical practice, it was too late for my grandmother.

Evolution and "We" Genes

Sometimes genes are expressed in certain regions of the world based on environmental conditions. For example, the disease thalassemia produces abnormal hemoglobin that causes a type of anemia; having this condition in a mild form is actually protection against malaria and is widely prevalent in parts of the world where this disease is endemic, such as South Asia and Africa.

In a major study, researchers from Oxford and Kenya studied the implications of alpha-thalassemia on children with malaria and diarrhea—both diseases cause the deaths of thousands of children in Africa.[10] They found thalassemia, with one or two α-globin genes lost, was associated with significant reductions in hospital admission rates caused by malaria, which is of great importance for the attempted development of malaria vaccines in the future.

Despite all the evidence linking salt and hypertension, we often hear people say, "My uncle ate a lot of salt, and he never developed high blood pressure," or that oft-quoted adage, "French women don't get fat." My father eats a lot of salt. At the family dinner table, we refer to him as "salt man" because of his liberal sprinkling of it on anything he is about to eat. His blood pressure has always been normal, and he is now in his eighties. Given this variability in our family history, I thought I'd test my daughter and myself to study our familial salt genes. Would she inherit her great-grandmother's blood pressure genes or her grandfather's salt safeguards?

The gene that regulates salt is the ACE gene, named after angiotensin-converting enzyme (ACE). ACE inhibitors are common medications used to lower blood pressure and reduce arterial disease. The ACE gene directs the body to produce the angiotensin-converting enzyme. We now know the risk variants of this gene, GA and AA—those who have these GA or AA variants of the ACE gene are at a greater risk of experiencing elevated blood pressure when they eat a lot of salt. People with the GG variant, a low-risk variant, do not exhibit this increased risk.

It turned out that I have the AA variant and need to ensure my salt intake is not too high (more details on the sodium content of foods in chapter 6); my daughter had a different variant, GA, which is also a high-risk variant. Being daddy's girl in this context meant there was no escape from genetic destiny.

I also have a normal variant of the CYP1A2 gene that relates to caffeine intake, but my daughter had an abnormal variant of that gene, which means that she needs to watch her coffee intake, or she can end up with heart disease. Genes like these coffee genes are the result of changes in human diets and experimentation—"we" genes.

As a species, our genetic blueprints became established as ancient humans migrated out of Africa on their own evolutionary walkabouts, conquering continents, discovering new diets, and it never occurred to them that as concepts of diet and diaspora emerged, so did new genes of our species. As we'll see in later chapters, marine and farming lifestyles brought with them different genetic baggage, as did other lifestyle changes over the millennia.

Life is about discoveries and creations, is it not? From friendships and new lands, animals and plants to technological advances and beautiful art in all its forms. Our genes respond to both our movements and our consumption. In the past fifty thousand years, evolution has progressed more rapidly than ever due to changes in our lifestyles.

Dean Ornish, clinical professor of the University of California, San Francisco, is a great believer in the power of lifestyle modification to influence genes. In a recent interview, he said:

J. Craig Venter has shown that one way you can change your genes is by making new ones. We are finding that another way you can change your gene expression is simply by changing your lifestyle . . . We found that changing [your] lifestyle actually changes gene expression. In only three months, we found that over five hundred genes were either up-regulated or down-regulated—in simple terms, turning on genes that prevent many chronic diseases, and turning off genes that cause coronary heart disease, oncogenes that are linked to breast and prostate cancer, genes that promote inflammation and oxidative stress, and so on.[11]

What Ornish and Venter found was that by changing our lifestyles, we can turn on good genes and turn off undesirable ones. We can be the change we want to see in our genetic footprint. Surely, we owe it to our next generation to make those changes.

Evolution and Drug Responses

The quest for wellness has inspired physicians in Western and Eastern medicine for thousands of years, but in recent times, the pace of life has made us look for chemical shortcuts. But before popping a pill, isn't it better to know what one's individual response is likely to be?

We saw earlier that the response to blood-thinning medications varies between individuals due to genetic differences. Understanding and personalizing drug treatment is especially important because our genetics may mean some drugs are ineffective for certain people. Indeed, genes even affect our responses to fake drugs.

Effective placebos are not a new concept and have been studied quite a bit. Ted Kaptchuk, who is a professor at Harvard Medical School, has focused his research on understanding the placebo effect. In one study, he divided migraine sufferers into three groups: one group received migraine medication, the second acupuncture, and the third a placebo. As expected, those on the migraine medication and the acupuncture improved, whereas those on the placebo did not. However, Kaptchuk's team had deliberately mixed things up—the real medication was the placebo, and the acupuncture needles were fake needles that did not penetrate skin, yet people got better!

Newer studies show that the ability of someone's mind to respond to healing by faith is genetically determined. Kaptchuk's team has now identified several genes that cause the placebo response. They've even come up with a new term for the study of genes and the placebo response: *the placebome*, a combination of *placebo* and *genome*.

The first placebo biomarker, the catechol-O-methyltransferase (COMT) gene, determines the extent of your placebo response—that is, you will be more likely to respond to drug-free or alternative therapies. A person with two copies of a variant of COMT has increased dopamine in the pre-frontal cortex of their brain. As we'll see in later chapters, the COMT gene influences the brain's levels of the neurotransmitter dopamine.

David Derbyshire wrote about acupuncture in *The Guardian*:

Despite more than three thousand studies into acupuncture since the 1970s, there is no evidence that any force resembling qi exists, or that it flows along invisible energy lines. The concept comes from a two-thousand-year-old misunderstanding of the human body and a culture that did not perform medical dissections . . . Just because qi is meaningless in the context of medical science doesn't mean acupuncture doesn't work.[12]

Reader Rx: Genetic Testing

If you are on medications such as blood thinners, antidepressants, antiepileptics, or diabetic or heart medications, it may be worth consulting your doctor about your individual genetic profile. It's probably easier and less expensive than you think. For my clients, I get these tests done via a saliva or blood sample, and we get the results in a few weeks. (At the end of the book there is information on a gene testing program I have developed that includes CYP2CP as well as dietary genes.) The important genes are CYP2D6, CYP3A4, and CYP2C9, with the latter especially important for those on blood thinners.

Key Points

. In the past fifty thousand years, we have entered a phase of rapid evolution due to diets and migration.
In genetics, there is a tradeoff between the individual and populations.
How you respond to a particular drug may be determined by your genes.
How you respond to non-drug therapies or placebos can also be determined by your genes.
People who respond to placebos also respond better to nurturing treatments such as bodywork or acupuncture.
Changing lifestyles actually changes your gene expression.
the future, personalized drug dosing based on genetics be the norm.

In the same article, Mark Bovey, president of the British Acupuncture Council, was quoted as saying, "Some patients get more benefit and some get less. The more useful thing is to look at the proportion of people who get a significant benefit."[13]

Charlotte Paterson, professor in Health Services Research at the University of Exeter, studied acupuncture in patients who had regularly attended a medical practice with symptoms and pain that could not be diagnosed by Western medical doctors.[14] They found patients felt much better and remained well for twelve months after acupuncture treatments. And the National Health Service in the UK has found that acupuncture reduces the cost of medical admissions—and has continued to fund this form of treatment as it has prevented costly hospitalizations.

The placebo effect and the COMT gene indicates that treatments that have not been proven in rigorous clinical studies, like energy healing, acupuncture, homeopathy, and so on, may work better in certain individuals. This isn't anything to be ashamed of—people with the high-dopamine allele of the COMT gene may do well on a placebo, although questions remain if this is nature or nurture. Reports suggest that people with these high-dopamine gene variants respond to nurturing treatments such as bodywork because they are generally more attuned to their environments or have more faith.[15] It isn't just the COMT gene. For example, alcoholics who had a high-dopamine producing allele of another gene, the DBH gene, showed less craving for alcohol when "treated" with a placebo drug rather than the conventional anti-craving agent, naltrexone. Ultimately it is the dopamine-dominance of a gene that determines the placebo or faith-healing response of an individual.

There are many drugs that show different responses due to particular gene variants, and if you are on any medications on the list below on a regular basis, it may be worth knowing if you have a gene variation, specifically a polymorphism.[16] Polymorphism is the occurrence of multiple alternative forms of a gene at the same chromosomal position; it allows natural selection to determine which trait survives. In some cases, gene polymorphisms may reduce a person's metabolic rate and increase plasma concentrations in the following drugs. In other words, if you have an abnormal variant of the genes listed below, your ability to metabolize certain medications will be affected:

CYP2D6 gene

Drugs affected:
    Antidepressants like amitriptyline, nortriptyline, imipramine,
        clomipramine
    Amphetamines
    Beta-blockers used for high blood pressure or heart conditions
    Tamoxifen, the breast cancer medication

CYP3A4 gene

Drugs affected:
    Sedatives like alprazolam, triazolam
    Antiepileptics like carbamazepine
    Psychiatric medications such as methadone, quetiapine,
        risperidone

CYP2C9 gene

Drugs affected:
    Blood thinners like warfarin
    Diabetic medications such as glipizide
    Antiepileptics such as phenytoin
    Anti-inflammatory drugs such as celecoxib or diclofenac

I have not provided an exhaustive list, as it isn't within the sco of this book, but it gives you an idea how gene testing can influ drug dosages in the future and that this is something worth di ing with your physician even now.

In fact, the future may be already here—the importance o drug variation was noted in 2005 in the FDA's approval o heart medication, a combination of a nitrate and a vasod mulated specifically for African American populations.

Conclusion

In the field of healthcare, we are faced with the between centralized national health systems a healthcare. The mapping of the genome and the ability of genetic testing have meant that, in the health programs can offer individualized nutrit based on one's genetics. But this requires an u the human race came from and our individu

After all, we are but one species of an the earth could not care less, for as m nological knowledge, it has come with environment. Isn't it strange that, as a s ical meetings to save our own enviro the (R$_X$)Evolutionary Road at night, ing about who should be driving.

Our entire human genome, ou has now been mapped, but such destination in mind. I do—a p enjoyed, where distractions of from healthy bodies, happy Ultimately, that's what health ecosystem where communi

2

THE SLUGGISH GENES: MOVE FOR YOUR BRAIN'S SAKE

Twins have a special claim upon our attention; it is that their history affords means of distinguishing between the effects of tendencies received at birth, and those that were imposed by the special circumstances of their after lives.

—Sir Francis Galton

Twins are always favorite study subjects when it comes to behavioral genetics. After all, if two people are genetically identical, surely it must follow that any change in behavior must be environmental?

The classical twin study design relies on studying twins raised in the same family environment, as this helps researchers look at the different inherited traits. A study in Finland actually looked at identical twins raised in similar surroundings—one who exercised and one who didn't.[1] In this study, which involved several pairs of adult twins, both twins had exercised as children, and their diets were the same. All that was different was that, as adults, one twin engaged in physical activity such as running and endurance exercise, but the other didn't.

What they found was mostly expected—the lazy twin weighed more, had more body fat, and had a higher risk of diabetes. However, what was even more significant was the effect endurance exercise had on the brain, especially in the parts of the brain associated with coordination and motor control. In short, not only did a few years of exercise make a huge difference in physical fitness, but it was also associated with significant brain changes that led to better brain fitness for daily life.[2]

Another research method often used is to compare identical and fraternal twins, because unlike fraternal twins with visible differences, identical twins are essentially genetic doppelgängers, and any changes to their behavioral or biological likeness can be attributed solely to the environment.

My editor for this book, Nevin, has a twin sister. I've been telling her that sluggish genes exist and could indicate a genetic predisposition toward laziness. Nevin reckons that she has to work harder than her sister to accomplish the same things, so she must have this Sluggish Gene. I'm waiting to run some tests on them to confirm.

Professor Wei Li of the Institute of Genetics and Developmental Biology (IGDB) in Beijing and Professor John Speakman, of the University of Aberdeen, collaborated on a search for what I have named the Sluggish Gene.[3] In studying overweight mice and obese patients, they came across a mutation in a gene called SLC35D3 and found that it produces a protein that plays a key signaling role in the brain's dopamine system. We know that when dopamine-related neurons in the brain are faulty, it leads to movement disorders such as Parkinson's disease. Normal cells have dopamine receptors on the surface, so the chemical can trigger some cells to initiate movement. In mice that had a faulty SLC35D3 gene, the dopamine receptors were trapped inside cells; therefore, these mice became couch potatoes. This finding not only is a key discovery in the search for a sluggish gene, but it also indicates a link between movement disorders and dopamine-related systems. When fat mice were treated with drugs that increased dopamine levels, they became more energetic and lost weight. Drug companies are now looking closely at the results of these studies and trying to develop new antiobesity pills.

Dopamine is an ancient neurotransmitter found in almost all animals. It has a relatively simple structure and is produced from the amino acid tyrosine. Dopamine is what I think evolution would call a *pleasure particle*, as it is related to positive-reinforcement behavior as well as opiate addiction.

In Fred Previc's book, *The Dopaminergic Mind in Human Evolution and History*,[4] he theorizes that increased levels of dopamine in the human body resulted due to an increase in meat consumption around two million years ago by primitive humans such as Homo habilis, and again increased around eighty thousand years ago due to the eating of fish oil, which has been shown to increase dopamine levels and reduces negative thoughts and depression. Previc believes we have become more and more used to higher and higher dopamine levels—and this has made our societies more manic, with higher intelligence, a sense of personal destiny, a religious or cosmic preoccupation, and an obsession with achieving goals.

Epigenetics is the study of changes in gene expression. To put it differently, it's the study of how genes can be turned on or off by certain factors without any change to the genetic code. Dopamine is a hub of epigenesis. When Emiliana Borrelli, a professor of microbiology and molecular genetics at the University of California, Irvine, was studying psychiatric disorders, she decreased dopamine release in rats by turning off midbrain dopamine receptors.[5] Astoundingly, almost two thousands genes in the prefrontal cortex were affected.

Dopamine, it seems, is what makes us modern humans tick. Its effects are everywhere in the brain, affecting thousands of genes, from excitement to romance, and from mania to movement. And if a mutant SLC35D3, one of the sluggish genes, fundamentally makes us stop moving, then surely it indicates that movement must be the primary purpose of the brain.

Movement Maketh the Brain

As Haruki Murakami writes, "I move, therefore I am"—no movement, no life.[6] That's not quite true if you ask a slumbering sloth. You should ask a sea squirt instead. These are fascinating creatures. The English neuroscientist Daniel Wolpert always uses the sea squirt as an example of why the brain evolved primarily for movement.

About 70 percent of our planet is seawater, so it is only natural that this constantly moving, majestic, and mellifluous body of liquid holds many secrets about our collective pasts. When we seek life on other planets, the first thing we look for is a sign of water. Even though the ocean is home to many unique and mysterious biological masterpieces, the sea squirt still remains one of my favorite creatures. This is an animal that has two life-forms—mobile and immobile. It begins life moving around on brightly colored, tentacle-like structures. Once it attaches itself to a rock, it begins to digest its brain, as the organ is redundant now. I said this in my recent TEDx Talk—if we find our rock and then spend our lives in front of a television, virtually immobile, we may as well eat our brains.[7] As Wolpert put it in his 2011 TED Talk:

So think about communication—speech, gestures, writing, sign language—they're all mediated through contractions of your muscles. So it's really important to remember that sensory, memory, and cognitive processes are all important, but they're only important to either drive or suppress future movements. There can be no evolutionary advantage to laying down memories of childhood or perceiving the color of a rose if it doesn't affect the way you're going to move later in life.[8]

Actually that's pretty logical because everything we do, we do because we move—for example, I am writing this book by moving many muscles: fingers typing on my computer keyboard, coffee-sipping lip muscles, eyebrows furrow as I consider this passage. Living life requires movement and, therefore, brain activity. Skin may sense touch, but without movement, our fingers or limbs cannot move toward an object we desire to touch. Movement is everything.

More and more, science points out that movement is not only essential, but it also actually makes our brains smarter in a kind of evolutionary feedback mechanism. In 2004, the evolutionary biologists Daniel E. Lieberman of Harvard and Dennis M. Bramble of the University of Utah published an article in the influential journal *Nature*, in which they hypothesized that our bipedal ancestors survived by becoming endurance athletes—by being able to chase and drag down prey.[9] Most other fast animals like cheetahs can run very fast in short bursts, but cannot run for a long time. They are sprinters, not endurance runners.

However, when humans became upright, everything about our bodies evolved to make us walk and run, two legged, over great distances. When compared to other primates, humans developed longer legs, shorter toes, less hair, and convoluted inner-ear mechanisms to maintain balance and keep us stable when we stand or run upright.

With this increase in movement, something else was happening, almost miraculously—our brains were becoming larger. The human brain is proportionally three times as big when compared to other animals' body size. In the beginning, people felt it was just because of increased movement. But increasingly, it appears endurance is also equally important. Dogs and rats, for example, are good endurance runners also, and these creatures also have larger-than-average brain sizes in proportion to their body sizes. Lieberman's team specifically decided to test the importance of endurance. They compared mice that were trained at endurance running with standard mice, and they found that, after a few generations, the mice that had undergone these fitness workouts had activated new genes and had innately high levels of substances that promote tissue growth and health, especially a protein called brain-derived neurotrophic factor (BDNF). BDNF is in humans too, and it not only makes your endurance better, but it also drives brain growth. The phrase "jogging your memory" may indeed be more literal than we imagine.

The Lieberman study was followed by a study by David A. Raichlen, an anthropologist at the University of Arizona.[10] He suggests the link between endurance exercise, especially leg movements, and the brain is thus: when an animal undertakes endurance exercise, they produce more BDNF in muscles. These muscles produce so much BDNF that some of this protein eventually ends up in the brain. The Canadian American cognitive scientist Steven Pinker's writings often suggest that evolution is a sneaky component in any study of psychology. Therefore, if humans developed endurance to hunt prey, and thereby developed larger brains, this was also because they were growing their ability to think and better plan tracking prey—an evolutionary game of chess that fed both body and brain.

Speaking of chess, I met the Russian chess champion Garry Kasparov at THiNK, an ideas conference, when we were at a book signing together. Garry was signing copies of *How Life Imitates Chess: Insights into Life as a Game of Strategy* and I was autographing copies of my previous book *Skin: A Biography*. That was the biggest book-signing I've ever had to do at one event—250 copies one after another. We discussed chess and his battles with the IBM supercomputer Deep Blue. Garry felt that a human is always superior to a computer, even though computers were getting better. When I asked him if it was a lack of concentration that made him lose to a computer once, he replied in the negative—it was because he had forgotten to play like a human, full of impulse and irrationality. He was trying to best the computer in a memory game and got beaten. But it was something else he said that got me thinking: "If I were sitting in front of a chess board, moving solid chess pieces about, the computer would have never beaten me." I'm not sure if Kasparov meant this, but therein is the answer, I reckon—to move chess pieces, we have to move many muscles, and this movement also makes our brain smarter. Daniel Wolpert would agree heartily. Wolpert says that it takes years to train a robot to pour a glass of water into different-sized cups, something a small child can master quickly. As long as we are moving something, the brain will do what it has to do much more efficiently and elegantly.

Evolution of Movement

Life evolved underwater, and in my view, this very fact suggests the importance of movement. Think of a society of primitive creatures evolving in stagnant water, and it doesn't seem very attractive. Perhaps life and water were always meant to be free flowing, always moving, like rivers, streams, underwater vents, and oceans. If we stop to think about it, creatures that seem still in water or space are not really immobile. As Vera Nazarian, a sci-fi writer, elegantly describes this phenomenon in *The Perpetual Calendar of Inspiration*:

> While everything else flits abut, the important things remain in place. Their stillness appears as reverse motion to our perspective, as relativity resets our motion sensors. It reboots us, allowing us once again to perceive.
> And now that we do see, suddenly we realize that those still things are not so motionless after all. They are simply gliding with slow individualistic grace against the backdrop of the immense universe.[11]

For the first 1.5 billion years of our planet, all creatures were single celled. Even these creatures were capable of movement and developed abilities to sense nutrients and other cells. Many of the components needed to transmit electrical signals and to receive chemical messages were present in these single-celled choanoflagellates. So, from the very beginning, creatures had the ability to communicate with others using a primitive nervous system, though not always for others' benefit. For example, primitive cnidarians (creatures like box jellyfish and some starfish), some of the earliest multicellular creatures, have specialized stinging cells that secrete a toxin to immobilize small prey. If creatures needed to fight as well as flee, sting, or avoid being stung, they needed to sharpen their ability to move, and this brought with it the need for muscles.

In 2010, the Royal Society's journal reported the finding of muscle tissue in an ancient cnidarian from a fossil dating to the Ediacaran Period, around 635 to 541 million years ago.[12] This was the first time muscle tissue had been discovered in a cnidarian. These organisms had eyes, a nervous system, and receptors, and the finding of muscle tissue raises an important chicken-or-the-egg question: does the brain control muscle or movement?

When I studied medicine, especially individual muscles and their nerve supplies, I struggled with the relevance of it all. Why did we have to memorize the different muscles within different compartments of the legs when many muscles were controlled by the same nerves or had overlapping functions? Why could we not just study movement instead? It seemed so much more practical. But education can often be impracticable, designed to find out what you don't know rather than how much you have understood. There were so many elements to remember: femoral or sciatic nerve, flexor or extensor, invertors or evertors—all these things ended up in my ultimately titanic memory.

When studies have been done on the muscles that control horizontal eye movements—lateral and medial rectus muscles, which are controlled in the abducens and oculomotor nuclei of the brain—researchers found that the brain does not appear to control motor units or antagonist muscles independently, but rather provides a framework, essentially acting like a soundless conductor, a hissing orchestral movement monitor that not only directs our motor systems on what to do, but also how to do it. Ultimately the brain controls both muscles *and* movement, acting as a nondictatorial choreographer of our lives.

The Taung Child was an infant who lived about 2.5 million years ago and whose remains were found at a quarry near Taung, in South Africa. The Taung Child was an australopithecine, an early species of hominid that developed all the muscles and bone structures needed to be bipedal. It is still debated whether they were exclusively two legged, and this may indeed be one of the reasons why this species did not survive, whereas our species, Homo sapiens, still endures today.

The Taung Child had a partially fused metopic suture of the skull; in other words, its pattern of brain development was similar to humans. Why did walking upright on two legs increase brain size? One viewpoint is that it freed up the forelimbs to do more complex hand tasks; further, standing tall also made us see more, and therefore, the visual areas of the brain increased. When Evan Eichler and colleagues looked at the evolution of human neural SRGAP2 gene, they found that it caused the development of the human cerebral cortex and that humans are the only species in which this gene was repeatedly duplicated.[13] The last major gene duplication took place two to three million years ago, a period when humans began first walking upright. Everything points to the evolutionary importance of being upright.

As evolution's grand plan progressed, humans grew enamored of their larger brain, one that furthered their ability to think, dance, and draw. Yet these early people did not comprehend nature's grand design, because nature may have the grandest designs, but part of the deal is that she always gets to keep the drawings. People were now busy foraging for food, fighting off competitors for a mate, festooning their caves, and finding playmates. All these caused an increase in brain size fundamentally due to the activity involved. If we stop to think about this, the brain in general has three "general purpose" movements: locomotion (e.g., walking, running, swimming), orienting (e.g., balancing or avoiding something by turning the head away), and grasping (either using the mouth or limbs). And every movement we make has an element of each of these actions. Muscles are elaborate, clumsy contraptions, yet the movements that a group of muscles coordinate are existentially elegant. You only need to observe a robot to understand this fact.

Imagine running to catch a bus or reaching for a pen (I know, writing is such hard work!). Previously, the way to understand the neural connections involved was to electrically stimulate these muscles. However, we know many muscles are activated and also many senses that help us accurately reach the target and avoid obstacles. So rather than studying individual muscles—the stuff I used to hate—the latest approach is brain mapping. Analyzing electrocorticography (think EKG for the brain) in epileptic patients who had had electrodes implanted in their brains, researchers were able to accurately map and reproduce upper and lower limb movements. Interestingly, when they tried the same for speech, they found a low sensitivity, indicating what we've been saying all along: the primary function of the brain is movement, not muscle contraction.

The idea of the brain being the organ of movement is a very recent one. Hippocrates thought that the brain was the seat of all intelligence, while Aristotle believed that to be the heart. During the time of Hippocrates, Greeks viewed the body as sacred and did not perform anatomical dissections or autopsies, and therefore, it was left to Galen—who, during the Roman Empire, began dissecting sheep, monkeys, dogs, and other animals—to understand anatomy. Galen sagely observed that, as the cerebellum was densely packed, it must be the controller of movement, while the softer cortex was the sensory part of the brain.

Of course, evolution of a larger brain meant that there was a trade-off. Walking two-legged meant humans ended up with smaller pelvises and thus found it difficult to accommodate a larger head during childbirth. Human babies have immature brains that are only a third of adult size, as they had to emerge from women who had begun walking upright and therefore had smaller pelvises—leading to the ultimate development of a new occupational species, wealthy obstetricians. During the first year of life, the brain almost doubles its weight, mostly in the cerebellum, which controls automatic movements and also coordinates the perception of senses. Should the cerebellum not develop properly, the child ends up with floppy muscles and clumsy movements.

There are several theories as to why movement is important. Standing upright increases heat to the head, and the need to dissipate this heat led to an increased blood supply to the brain. However, we know that merely increasing blood supply does not do the job alone. The brain also has a pacemaker or clocklike function that allows it to turn muscles on or off to conserve power. However, since these oscillations occur forty times per second—rather like a movie in multiple frames—we do not notice any discontinuity or jerkiness in our muscle movements. If the head merely needed to be upright, why did humans adopt a two-legged walk? They could have simply sat two legged like a Buddha of evolution.

For a start, standing made our range of vision greater, and therefore, taller, upright humans had an advantage over others in locating predators. We must remember this was a time filled with danger, with many predators competing for prey. Man's footprint on the planet was small, and he had to fight for survival and territory. It filled his thoughts and determined his actions: fear, fight, flight, and, eventually, freedom.

Most animals stand on their hind legs when they fight, offering them not just the illusion of height but also improved punching power. David Carrier from the University of Utah actually tested this hypothesis by measuring the force and energy produced when human subjects struck objects in postures—standing, kneeling, sitting, crouched like apes, and so on.[14] The primary attack weapons of primates are their jaws and large canine teeth. Darwin shrewdly observed that these canines shrank as people began to walk upright, at which point their forelimbs became their attack weapons. Carrier noted that for all types of striking—downward, upward, side and forward punches—being on two legs nearly doubled the force generated. There is a proverb in the slums of India that says that once you leave a mother's womb, you better learn to fight—or crawl back in and cower. This may be an evolutionary truism.

Francis Bacon once wrote, "Histories make men wise; poets, witty; the mathematics, subtle; natural philosophy, deep; moral, grave; logic and rhetoric, able to contend."[15] The evolution of movement was like that—nature decided to use neither mathematics nor art but logic. First, there was random movement, then came purposeful activity. As man ran longer distances, his brain became both bigger and wiser, and chemicals such as dopamine brought him the ability to dare, dream, dispute, and draw. Ultimately, nature used science, which may seem a blunt tool to some, lazy with its poetry and philosophy, but the gradual evolution of movement was essentially common sense at its best.

Gravity, Muscle Movement, and Muscle Development

Given that we have just discussed how movement has determined the evolution of brain development, it follows that we should ask: does restriction of movement reduce brain function? Is muscle movement still relevant as humans become more stationary? After all, we live in an era when humans are at their most sedentary—and as Mark Twain once said in jest: "I'm pushing sixty years of age . . . and that's enough exercise for me."[16] Even when we are sedentary, gravity is relentlessly at work. Life on earth means that gravity is our constant companion, one we cannot shake off easily. J. B. S. Haldane once described gravity thus:

> Gravity, a mere nuisance to Christian, was a terror to Pope, Pagan, and Despair. You can drop a mouse down a thousand-yard mine shaft; and, on arriving at the bottom, it gets a slight shock and walks away, provided that the ground is fairly soft. A rat is killed, a man is broken, a horse splashes.[17]

Confucius once said, "Gravity is only the bark of wisdom's tree, but it preserves it."[18] One thing worth bearing in mind is that all creatures on earth evolved under the conditions imposed by gravity, and there is no escaping this fact. Therefore, when astronauts go into space, due to their confined environment and lack of gravity, they end up moving less than on earth and studies have shown that BDNF, the protein we discussed earlier that's responsible for growth and survival of neurons, gets affected. This BDNF is produced by both bone and muscle during exercise, confirming both the importance of movement for life and that, during inactivity, some parts of the brain fail to mature or develop properly. People suffering from depression or Parkinson's disease also have lowered BDNF, indicating a link to the chemical dopamine, which is depleted in the brain cells of people with Parkinson's disease.

It transpires that we have an important protein called AMP-activated protein kinase (AMPK) that gets turned on during exercise. Genes that make these proteins enable muscles to make more energy from sugars by having more mitochondria, the energy-making powerhouses of each cell. Given that mice that lack these genes have both lower numbers of mitochondria as well as defective AMPK in their muscles, scientists could surmise that the two were linked. Gregory

Steinberg of McMaster University ran a study on mice with and without genes for AMPK: the ones with normal genes were typical mice that ran and scurried about a lot; the ones with the defective AMPK genes were couch-potato mice. The maximum they could manage was the length of a room.

Herein lies the crux of the problem: our lifestyle has repercussions. If we spend a lot of time doing nothing with the muscles we can control, especially our arms and legs, we end up with lower levels of mitochondria, and therefore, it is much harder to get going again, as lowered levels of mitochondria come with lower AMPK. Lack of movement results in us developing another one of these sluggish genes. As Steinberg put it:

> When you exercise, you get more mitochondria growing in your muscle. If you don't exercise, the number of mitochondria goes down. By removing these genes [that control AMPK], we identified the key regulator of the mitochondria is the enzyme AMPK . . . As we remove activity from our lives due to emerging technology, the base level of fitness in the population is going down and that is reducing the mitochondria in people's muscles. This, in turn, makes it so much harder for people to start exercising.[19]

That passage alone delivers a stern scientific message to all couch potatoes.

Movement has been an important part of almost all life-forms, but when and why did we develop muscles? Historically, scientists have believed that animals evolved during the Cambrian Period around 540 million years ago. In the preceding Ediacaran Period, which spanned from about 580 million to 541 million years ago, researchers had believed that the earth consisted of mainly fungi and plants—until recently. But that's the problem with prehistoric nostalgia. For every dinosaur or mammoth bone found, there's a fossil lurking inside a rock somewhere, waiting to disprove a theory.

In 2014, a fossilized creature was found in Canada—this creature was a relative of sea anemones and jellyfish and was found to contain muscle tissue. This caused great excitement, and the fossil was duly installed in the evolutionary hall of fame by classifying it as a new genus and species: Haootia quadriformis. This finding showed that once animals moved beyond being mere sponges, they needed muscles to roam, reproduce, and run from danger. Further, the time frame this occurred in caused a rethink of the evolutionary time line for the development of more complex creatures.

One of the ways to understand the brain-muscle axis is to analyze metabolomes—the total number of byproducts of metabolism, such as calcium or water, found in these bodily tissues. When researchers at Shanghai's CAS-MPG Partner Institute for Computational Biology and Germany's Max Planck Institute compared the metabolomes of humans and chimpanzees, they found that human brains had evolved fourfold, but human muscle had evolved tenfold.[20] However, when they tested the muscular strength of humans against apes, they found humans to be much weaker. These researchers wrote:

> We hypothesize that metabolic evolution of human muscle and brain metabolomes may have occurred in parallel. Studies demonstrating a connection between aerobic exercise and cognitive performance in humans of different age indicate that these two organs might be metabolically related. Furthermore, it was also previously suggested that rescaling of energetically expensive organs, such as the gut, allowed the development of a larger brain in human evolution.[21]

What these researchers and other evolutionary biologists now agree on is that we developed larger brains at the expense of muscles.

There was an evolutionary trade-off. To boost our brains, our muscle strength was sacrificed, and this explains the metabolic and genetic link between muscle activity and the brain. Therefore, the types of exercises that boost brains are those that involve muscle movement and endurance, not sheer brute strength. You are not going to gain brain fitness by pumping iron, but dancing might help you.

The Surprising Benefits of Dance

Recently, scientists discovered a new muscle enzyme, SIRT3, that is involved in fat metabolism and energy production. This enzyme belongs to a group of proteins called sirtuins that are thought to be responsible for both muscle health and longevity. Sirtuins are now thought to be key players in increasing longevity and decreasing metabolic diseases. Some sirtuins like SIRT3 are located inside mito-chondria of human skeletal muscle. Wait a minute, you say. If our brains evolved by weakening our muscles, creating dancers rather than defenders, can dancing make us live longer?

Friedrich Nietzsche once wrote, "I would only believe in a God who knew how to dance."[22] As a philosopher he must have seen some deep meaning in dance—a movement that is multilayered and provides an opportunity for different interpretations; it is aerobic articulation for the cognitive mind.

The concern when it comes to dancing for our cerebral health and longevity is that only some of us are natural dancers. It doesn't have anything to do with creativity. I think I am creative, but put me on a dance floor, and arrhythmic spasms are the only way to describe my moves in literal terms. Still, if I started dancing, would I live longer?

I put this question to associate professor Dr. Dafna Merom from the Western Sydney University (WSU) School of Science and Health. Merom has studied nearly fifty thousand people and concluded that dancing can halve your risk of heart disease, but there's a caveat—

you need to begin before age forty. Merom, who found that dance was a superior form of exercise to walking, states: "Some styles of ballroom or folk dancing almost mimic the short bouts of vigorous intensity we see in interval training."[23] Interval training is a method of exercise where series of low- to high-intensity exercises are alternated with periods of rest. Studies have shown that interval training increases maximal oxygen uptake—the measure of oxygen that we can use. In effect, one develops endurance in intervals rather than by continuous training.[24]

When I studied people living in the blue zones of the health world—ageless places where many folk live significantly longer lives than people in other parts of the world—I was interested in why so many of these were located on islands: the Greek island of Ikaria, Okinawa in Japan, and Sardinia in Italy. What made islands different? Does the isolation reduce infection rates, or is the secluded geography a mere coincidence?

Perhaps islands merely possess an allure and tempt us to escape to them because even though water is everywhere, nowhere else is our encirclement so obvious. One may as well be floating on the sea of time—a place where memories and family stories remain unspoiled. A few years ago, I read the story of Stamatis Moraitis, a Greek war veteran from the island of Ikaria who came to America for medical treatment toward the end of the Second World War. Moraitis eventually moved to Florida and lived the American dream—condo, children, and a Chevy. In 1976, during the bicentennial year of America's founding, Moraitis went to see a doctor, as he had begun to feel short of breath and struggled to climb stairs. After investigations and a multitude of medical opinions, he was given the diagnosis terminal lung cancer. Essentially, he was told to go home to die, as his illness was expected to prove fatal within a year.

Moraitis felt that it was perhaps wise to go back to the Greek island of Ikaria, where his ancestors were buried in oak-laden cemeteries overlooking the green-blue waters of the Aegean Sea. Ikaria is an island of roughly one hundred square miles and approximately one hundred people per square mile. People there live the simple life—eat minimal meat, nap a lot, stay up late, and eat lots of olives and vegetables. And their social connections are very strong—communities gather in the evenings to philosophize, play dominoes, and dance. Dance. At night, well past bedtimes in the West, people move dining tables to the corner of the room, link their arms, and dance to traditional Greek music.

Moraitis's story received much attention in America and ended up the subject of a documentary because he ended up living much longer than predicted—not a year longer, or a decade longer, but he even made a trip back to America twenty-five years after he first moved to Ikaria purely to figure out why he had lived so long. When Dan Buettner of the *New York Times* interviewed Moraitis in 2012, he couldn't help asking Moraitis what his doctors had made of his surviving lung cancer, especially since as many as nine physicians had given him less than a year to live.[25] Moraitis responded that he didn't have the answers, as his "doctors were all dead" by the time he had returned to America.

Buettner ended up establishing a consultancy to investigate these hotspots, or blue zones, of healthiness, where people lived much longer than their peers, and he wrote a book about places like Ikaria and Okinawa, both well-known blue zones.[26] This led to a flurry of research into longevity, as if it were a medical condition that needed curing.

Medicine derives from the Latin word *medicus*, which means physician; *physician*, in turn, derives from *physica*, which means "things related to nature." Therefore, is the quest for longevity really medicine? Aren't birth and death perfectly natural? Isn't a scientific life, after all, a quest for answers? Perhaps as medicine has become more of an industry than a vocation, people have sought far and wide for places where people live longer, seemingly forever, in an attempt to tap those resources for industry and inventions.

There have been several other locations whose claims for longevity didn't stack up on closer scrutiny—Pakistan's Hunza Valley or Ecuador's Vilcabamba Valley. Neither were islands and the former was especially noted for its lack of dancing. But when medical researchers looked closely, it was clear that most of their residents simply didn't know their ages, and birth certificates were virtually nonexistent. But one place that had meticulous *koseki* (family registry) records and Methuselah-like defiance of mortality was the island of Okinawa, Japan. This led to the groundbreaking Okinawa Centenarian Study that looked at what made this island special.[27] First, researchers investigated whether there was a particular longevity gene. Thus far, even though there was no apparent genetic magic bullet for permanence, there was a higher incidence of the apolipoprotein E (ApoE) gene—a gene that is related to exceptional longevity that seems to be especially common among these dancing islanders. And when people over the age of one hundred in Okinawa were studied, the calculation of how important genes might be to their condition (of extreme age) showed a (likelihood or "risk" of siblings becoming centenarians) factor of 6.5 (in contrast, among Utah centenarians in America, it is 2.3), indicating the strong genetic component for lifespans in Okinawa.

There might be other factors at play here, such as diet or marine air, but we now know this much is true: in blue zones, dancing seems to be part of regular activity. Okinawa is actually referred to as the "islands of performing arts," as people there enjoy music and dancing—either *Koten buyo*, a more traditional dance, or *Zou odori*, which is rather like folk opera.

Professor Richard P. Ebstein of Hebrew University's Scheinfeld Center for Human Genetics in the Social Sciences has spent several years studying different groups of dancers.[28] Both dancers and athletes showed different variants of genes that coded for a serotonin transporter and an arginine vasopressin receptor (1a), further showing that, as human brains evolved, our muscles became weaker but more attuned for movements such as dancing.

Arginine vasopressin receptor (1a) is known to be a big player in social communication and bonding behaviors—things that helped our ancestors survive the last ice age. Both are elements in the human social expression of dancing. Ebstein's team concluded that specific genes—AVPR1a and SLC6A4—are associated with creative dance performance. This may explain why Africans are natural dancers—although we haven't done population studies to confirm this—and it may be no accident they were descendants of the earliest human colonies.

I must confess that I read his paper with some relief. I've always known that my crappy dancing was not due to a lack of effort—my flesh was willing, but my genetic die had been long since cast. Still, there is some hope. Dancing helps the brain, but evolutionary biology does not demand technical perfection, even if the craft and the cranium seem discordant.

However, the problem with the genome being mapped is that we want unwavering conclusions from genetics so we can have either an answer or reveal some kind of hidden destiny. But the problem with scientific methods and the intricacies of gene expression is that they both leave some wiggle room—sometimes genes are activated and at other times they remain sleepers, so we are still investigating.

Until now, we've been looking at the benefits of dance and movement on brain development, but can dancing actually reduce the risk of brain diseases like Parkinson's or dementia?

When electroencephalograms (EEGs) of different people were studied, the brain tracings revealed increased activation in the theta (4–8 Hz), alpha (8–13 Hz), and beta (13–20 Hz) spectral bands, and higher mean frequency in the delta (0.25–4 Hz), theta, and beta bands in more active individuals, indicating that being physically fit activates the brain and improves cognitive functions.[29]

In a small but significant study, Dr. Paul Dougall at the University of Strathclyde in Scotland studied a group of seventy Scottish dancers and compared this group with others that performed conventional exercises like walking, golf, and swimming.[30] Dougall concluded that dancers were more agile, had stronger legs, and could walk more briskly than those performing other exercises. Celtic dances, like traditional Scottish and Irish dancing, typically involve a lot of leg movements, and since becoming upright and two legged is what differentiated modern man, these dances tend to outperform other exercise when it comes to improving brain function.

In Oliver Sacks's book *Awakenings*, largely about Parkinson's disease, he noted:

> Patients so affected find that as soon as they "will" or intend or attempt a movement, a "counter-will" or "resistance" rises up to meet them. They find themselves embattled, and even immobilized, in a form of physiological conflict—force against counter-force, will against counter-will, command against countermand.[31]

Parkinson's seems a dreadful disease, determined to take from us our freedom and mechanize our movement—something terrible for terrestrial lives. Assistant professor at Emory University's Division of General and Geriatric Medicine Madeleine Hackney also holds a BFA in dance and has researched its effects on people with Parkinson's disease and specifically compared different dance types against exercises like Tai Chi, which have shown to reduce falls in the elderly.

A few years ago, she ran a study with seventy-five patients of Parkinson's disease attending twenty lessons of tango, waltz/foxtrot, and Tai Chi and compared their movement against those who had no therapy.[32] Hackney studied the effects of these interventions against Health Related Quality of Life (HRQoL)—essentially, medical jargon for a patient's assessment of the impact their illness has on their normal life. What her team found was interesting—waltz/foxtrot, Tai Chi, or "no intervention" had no benefit, but tango did.

The tango is a tempestuous dance. It has many guises, the Argentinians say—the mask of intimacy as dancers hold each other close, the mask of secrecy as the upper bodies are still, and the mask of wild abandon as the legs entwine again and again in a passionate duel. But more importantly, if you do it in true Argentinian style, unlike most ballroom dances, it typically does not have predetermined movements. You go where your partner or the music takes you, effectively making your improvisations reflect your feelings or the music. This was actually why people with Parkinson's disease did well in Hackney's study—or, indeed, why the traditional dances of Ikaria and Okinawa are so helpful. People performing the waltz or foxtrot rely on memory of specific foot movement, whereas tango relies on working closely with a partner in the moment. Thus, exercises with predetermined positions like yoga or Tai Chi and foot movements such as the foxtrot could still be beneficial for breathing, cardiac fitness, and agility, but specifically partnered dances like the tango or Celtic dances, where leg movements are predominant, had the greatest benefit when it comes to reducing dementia or improving movement disorders such as Parkinson's disease. As I said to the audience when I was at the Dalkey Book Festival in Dublin—we can even forgive the Irish for *Riverdance*!

Dancing and its benefits can even start before birth. In 2015, scientists at Institut Marquès in Barcelona studied the effects of music on fetuses of between fourteen and thirty-nine weeks. They used an intra-vaginal music system (which they called a "babypod") and filmed the ultrasound scans of babies "listening" to music.[33] We know that at around sixteen weeks of pregnancy, babies develop their hearing abilities, but astonishingly, these babies began to open their mouths and also move their legs to the music—these dancing fetuses were recorded on ultrasound scans that show these unborn babies responding to the music. Dr. Marisa López-Teijón, who led the study, was quoted as saying that the findings show a fetus responds to music by moving its mouth and tongue "as if they were trying to speak or sing." The fetal origin hypothesis suggests this fetal dance may help brain development later. After all, fetal life is a hotbed of neuroplasticity—the baby's brain triples in weight during the last trimester of pregnancy and the surface area of the cerebellum, the part of the brain that coordinates movements during activities like dancing, increases thirtyfold.

I mentioned earlier in this chapter that the fundamental reasons for the existence of movement were threefold: locomotion (e.g., walking), orienting (e.g., balance or avoiding something) and grasping—all things that develop early in childhood. The reason the tango is better for the brain than all other forms of dance is because it specifically involves training in all three areas. Argentine tango dancers are taught a specific technique of walking backward; they must also be aware of their surroundings and avoid bumping into other people, especially during street tango dances. Tango involves movements like *enganche*, where a leg or foot is used to wrap a partner in a hook or a grasp. In studies where research looked at a patient's ability to get up and mobilize, especially in those with movement disorders such as Parkinson's disease, researchers found that what they term timed up-and-go (TUG) was improved.[34] People in tango groups decreased TUG time by two seconds, while waltz/foxtrot showed no change in TUG time and Tai Chi improved TUG time by one second.

Dancing actually dates back to the earliest times when humans became upright and began to walk two legged, further indicating its evolutionary importance as both a social and a physical activity. Ward and others date the earliest practice of dance to two million years ago, to earlier species of now-extinct hominids.[35]

Wondering if the reason dancing outperforms virtually every other exercise modality, including postural exercises like Tai Chi, is due to walking on two legs, researchers put people through MRI and PET scans while simulating dancing, especially those involving leg movements.[36] This particular study conducted positron emission tomography (PET) scans while amateur dancers performed small-scale, bipedal dance steps on an inclined surface in an attempt to not only localize the parts of the brain involved, but also understand the relation to music and metrics. When the researchers studied these scans of dance movements and linked them to metric rhythms, there was far more activity on these scans when compared to non-metric rhythms, leading them to conclude that dance, as a universal human activity, involves a complex combination of processes related to the patterning of bipedal motion, a fundamentally human method of locomotion. Maybe this is why the tango translates to brain fitness—because it's a walk as much as a dance; as much as it is formal and pretty, the movements are unconditional and resigned, creating intense consultations between our brains and other arbiters of movement in our bodies.

As Chuck Fishman said in an episode of the TV series *Early Edition*:

> We enter this world alone. We leave it pretty much the same way. And in between, a dance we call life. Problem is it takes two to tango. So we look for signs; something to help us to find our perfect partners: a smile, a wave. But we have to be careful, because while some signs can be misinterpreted, others can be missed completely... Some dances you sit out. Others you change partners. The important thing is ... you never stop dancing.[37]

When I started writing this chapter about the evolutionary biology of movement and brain development, I imagined that I'd be writing more about yoga, Pilates, Tai Chi, and that kind of stuff, not dance. But the pursuit of scientific facts brings fascinating revelations.

A scientific life is after all an individual opera—and each of us has our own tango to lead.

Tomorrow Never Comes

My father is a retired surgeon. He grew up in a family of nine, the son of a Lutheran church minister. After completing his surgical training in India, he worked as a consultant surgeon in England before my parents decided to return to India, where our roots are, to pursue medical mission work. Strategically, it was an unequal trade-off—leaving assured National Health Service incomes and pensions for a cash-deprived experiment caring for those with health needs that had never been measured. This was India at its poorest, full of social dislocation, caste exploitation, and stoic endurance when faced with lack of water or food. We were in such small towns that at one stage, I used to go to school in an ox cart.

Certainly we had none of the money that other doctors in private hospitals made. Only years later, when worried about how they would fund their children's private-school education, did my father end up dabbling in private practice. My overriding memory of childhood is of being around hospital wards: the smell of formalin and phenol; patients lying on wrought-iron beds, painted white, carefully arranged so that no one's feet pointed to a door (people in south India believe that only corpses lie with their feet facing the door).

The operating rooms were ones that I had no access to until I was older and an apprentice surgeon, a medical student. Ever since, operating theater beds have held an allure for me—I have two antique ones—rather like metallic islands where bits of tissue or organs are put together again, where hope raises its head and tries to look beyond the oversize light that hangs from the ceiling.

Perhaps there is a touch of voyeurism in our fascination with surgery. For over twenty years, my father and mother tended to the health of others. Patients were plentiful; vacations were rare. Anyone who came received care, and those who could pay the meager fees, paid. It was that kind of hospital—educational, compelling, and smug in its socialism. Many babies born there were named after my parents; the willing incarceration of a highly trained surgeon in a mission hospital was sometimes pitied and sometimes envied.

Sometimes your memory takes a picture and then etches it into the recesses of your brain. I remember my father hunched over an operating table, using his gloved hands to fix broken people. When I look back over photographs from those days, in each of those images, I can see him getting increasingly bent over, stooped due to a wrecked back from all that operating. Physically, the work was demanding and had become a physical burden and a mental morass, yet it ruled his life and fulfilled him.

Once my parents retired, we got to spend time together. Except it was now my turn to be busy.

When one begins to lose one's memory it happens so gradually that it takes time to realize. Last year, at the age of eighty-three, my father began to lose his short-term memory. In the beginning, I thought it was just benign forgetfulness. The first person to really figure out that his memory was failing was our dog, Zack, as he realized he could get fed twice. Zack began to follow my father closer and closer. The celebrated author Terry Pratchett wrote this in a blog about dementia:

Each person who lives with one of these diseases will be affected in uniquely destructive ways. I, for one, am the only person suffering from Terry Pratchett's posterior cortical atrophy which, for some unknown reason, still leaves me able to write—with the help of my computer and friend— bestselling novels. There's no clearly plotted pathway to the course of these diseases.[38]

It is like that for Dad. One day, he'd simply forget he'd already had coffee with me; another day, he'd get disorientated in a crowd and begin walking the wrong way. One inevitable fantasy for any family affected by someone losing their memory is that we can reverse all the pathologies. Dad can remember events during the Second World War and his time in England, explain complex surgical operations in the finest detail, but not what he had for breakfast today. My mother, hoping to prevent any embarrassment among strangers, has gradually begun to run his conversations. Memory loss and dementia are scary conditions, especially as we cannot see the enemy, let alone remember his name.

Do to the years spent in operating theaters, my father's body is much the worse for wear and stiff. If he lies on the floor, his head cannot touch the ground. No one had told him about stretching or the importance of being supple. If we need to look after our bodies before our memories deteriorate, we need to learn from the sea squirt—move, dance the tango, stop our joints from seizing up.

Forgetfulness is in many ways a positive thing, as it is often accompanied by its mate, freedom. I realized that, for Dad, content with life, leisure, and family, he needed the fun of forgetfulness as much as he needed the pleasure of remembrance.

For around 1.5 billion years, life-forms existed as single-celled creatures. As these creatures eventually decided to conglomerate into multicellular organisms, they needed cell adhesion molecules such as cadherins, and as higher organisms evolved, these cell adhesion molecules extended their family to incorporate things like integrins that act as scaffolding proteins. For a long time, these molecules were ignored by medicine, but starting around the early 1970s, people began to identify these molecules that caused cells to bond. Although we now know that cell adhesion molecules have an important evolutionary purpose, they can be double-edged tools. If you lack cadherins, clumps of cells could break off and clog your arteries or lymphatics, as happens in tumors. If you have an overproduction of cadherins, it can worsen joint stiffness and arthritis, as the joints end up too sticky. Increasingly, research shows that an overproduction of these cell adhesion molecules worsens conditions like rheumatoid arthritis.[39] Recent studies have shown that increased cell adhesion molecules like N-cadherins affect signaling pathways for mitogen-activated protein kinase (MAPK), a pathway related to cell division. MAPK is also implicated in Alzheimer's dementia.[40] Joints need to be loose and another reason why dancing helps the brain.

Procrastination vs. Sluggishness

In this chapter, we've been discussing why movement matters and the benefits of certain types of movement. But if evolution is all about evolving ourselves to the next level, why do we struggle with things that are good for us—endurance exercise, dancing, reducing sugar intake, and so on?

We've discussed many sluggish genes in the context of movement—if movement, especially two-legged activity and endurance exercise, is so important, why do we struggle to motivate ourselves to undertake such activity? Sluggishness is inherently bad for our brains, muscles, and lifespans, but as it transpires, procrastination may be good.

The word *procrastination* derives from the Latin *cras* for "tomorrow." Our species, Homo sapiens, migrated out of Africa one hundred thousand years ago; about fifty thousand years ago, a group of these original folk walked to Australia; and more recently, ten thousand to fifteen thousand years ago, people from Europe migrated into Asia. Neanderthals, a competing species of humans, hunkered down in Europe during the ice age but went extinct somewhere around twenty-eight thousand to forty thousand years ago. Neanderthals shared 99.5 percent of our DNA, and despite the fact

Homo sapiens have larger brains than Neanderthals, many scientists now believe that they were not less intelligent than us.[41] It turns out that our brain was larger not because we were more intelligent, but because we were better at complex planning. This, as we saw earlier, could be because we ended up the most upright of hominid species. However, complex planning is where procrastination ended up preserving our ancestral people.

As human beings, we are frail and ignorant and don't make efforts to preserve our surroundings or planet. The earth cannot escape us—it is stuck with our efforts at mining, fracking, chopping down trees, and our more subtle persecutions. As much as we have destroyed nature, it is important that we maintain a connection to and preserve the land that has been so bountiful for us, but we cannot comprehend this.

You see, nature and evolution look at the bigger picture with the understanding that the planet is sustainable, but Homo sapiens may not be. That's why evolution does not mold each individual into perfection but allows us the freedom to be individuals—because ultimately if we raze ourselves to the ground, a new species shall emerge.

On another note, while movement and venturing into the outdoors was good for our ancestors, life was fraught with risk and predators. Walking long distances helped the species develop a larger brain, but we also needed complex planning for survival. Planners survived; doers didn't always do so. That's the beauty of evolution—it plans things carefully. As species move to the top of the food chain or brain-size pyramid, it does not want to cause damage that puts the whole species at risk. So nature experiments with a few—the procrastinators.

Cal Newport, the assistant professor of computer science at Georgetown University, who specializes in the theory of distributed algorithms, has written about "the procrastinating caveman."[42] As he sees it, procrastination is not a character flaw but instead a finely tuned evolutionary adaptation. Procrastination is effectively our brain not

buying our plans, because they are either not thought through well enough or are doomed to fail. Newport talks about the three most common reasons people give when they put things off for another day: fear, perfectionism, and unfinished or poor-quality work. And Newport adds another to this list: the brain simply doesn't believe in your plan. As he says:

> Complex planning is a preverbal adaptation, so it's not going to manifest itself as a voice in your head exclaiming, "Plan rejected!" Instead, it's going to be more intuitive: a biochemical cascade designed to steer you away from a bad decision—something, perhaps, that feels like a lack of motivation to get started.
>
> If this explanation is true, then you would also expect that students with smart study habits to struggle less with procrastination. This is exactly what I observed when I studied elite undergrads . . . procrastination is not a character flaw but instead a finely-tuned evolutionary adaptation.[43]

If we stop to think about this, it makes complete sense. We can identify with those times we had a business plan that we had written up in great detail but were delaying doing something about—and if we were to be honest about it, either we were not ready or hadn't thought it through well enough. In Newport's words: "You shouldn't lament procrastination but instead listen to it."[44]

Newport and other scientists' similar hypotheses about procrastination being a biochemical evolutionary trait have now actually been proven by studies. MRI scans were done to assess resting-state functional connectivity (RSFC) between brain regions; essentially, RSFC is a measure of the connectivity of our neurons (i.e., how neuron activation in one part of the brain causes changes in another part). Examining the human brain as a network of functionally inter-

acting brain regions, rather than as anatomical lobes, has now given us great insights into large-scale neuronal communication. This is evolution at its finest, playing with our minds, challenging our science, informing us, and destroying our perceptions. As we saw earlier, movement matters more than muscle; likewise, connectivity matters in the brain rather than size alone. After all, men have 10 percent larger brains than females, but it doesn't make them more "wired" or smarter.

Studying MRI scans during rest can effectively tell you how wired you are. If your wiring is a bit awry, if your RSFC is reduced, the more you will procrastinate. A study looking into the predictability of procrastination found that procrastination was associated with reduced functional connectivity between brain areas involved in self-regulation.[45] In looking at the link between procrastination and the stress response, several studies also show that procrastination is strongly linked to stress symptoms and increases your risk of heart disease and hypertension.

Freud pondered procrastination and saw it as a means for delaying the inevitable—death—and any associated stress was a fight-or-flight response against Thanatos, the Greek god of death. Procrastination was seen as the thief of time, able to make off with valuable minutes, but now many psychologists believe that it may instead be a curator of creativity, incubating our many ideas long enough to allow the good ones to surface as creative solutions. If we were planning to charge and attack a wooly mammoth or a saber-toothed tiger, the procrastination gene made us come up with improved plans such as developing better spears and so forth.

Cedric Ginestet talks of "the unbearable lightness of procrastination" and explains it thus: "Procrastination always goes in the same direction, away from the tedious and toward the pleasant."[46] Viewed in this way, putting stuff off for another day becomes both a time- and energy-conserving strategy. Sloths, which are excellent swimmers,

although they are extremely slow on land, would agree—lack of movement and camouflage end up being useful to avoid detection. For sloths, both three toed and two toed, doing as little as you can may indeed be an evolutionary survival strategy.

In Chinese philosophy, yin and yang is the concept of competing forces—opposites that are interconnected and interdependent, challenging each other to greater heights. As Newton's third law states, for every action, there is an equal and opposite reaction. The other side of procrastination is impulsivity, where a creature does not plan but acts right away. As it transpires, even in genetics, the principle of complementary and contrary forces applies.

Daniel Gustavson of the University of Colorado Boulder and his colleagues studied twins—181 pairs of identical twins and 166 pairs of fraternal twins were analyzed in multiple studies and conclusions were made that procrastination and impulsivity are genetically linked, suggesting that the two traits stem from similar evolutionary origins.[47] Strangely, making rash decisions or failing to achieve goals both stem from a shared genetic foundation, indicating a degree of genetic Zen.

In the book *The Procrastination Equation*, Piers Steel wrote, "Without a genetic component, the ability to procrastinate couldn't easily be passed on. We evolved to be procrastinators."[48] So does a procrastinator propagate another procrastinator? Scientists often turn to twin studies to resolve such complex questions. In 1875, Sir Francis Galton wrote about such studies being an excellent way to conclude the nature versus nurture debate: "Twins have a special claim upon our attention; it is that their history affords means of distinguishing between the effects of tendencies received at birth and those that were imposed by the special circumstances of their after lives."[49] However, as I mentioned earlier, twin studies have remained controversial, as to be considered scientifically valid, both twins must have identical environments and be identical, rather than fraternal.

With the emergence of genomics and the ability to obtain universal DNA, we now have the ability to improve the quality of the assumptions we can make from these studies.

The rationale for using twins to study traits like procrastination runs like this:[50]

1. If procrastination is wired through evolution, it should be a hereditary trait like impulsivity (the latter has now been established in genetic studies).
2. If procrastination and impulsivity are linked (i.e., the former is a byproduct of the latter), the genetics of procrastination should be the same as that for impulsivity.
3. An individual's difficulty in managing goals should be explainable by these shared genetic variations.

How can the same gene end up producing opposite effects? This is actually known as the "French flag model" and has to do with concentrations of the morphogen. A *morphogen* is a molecule that acts directly on cells to produce specific cellular responses depending on its local concentration. At some concentrations of these morphogens, genes tend to cause a particular effect; at different concentrations, they do the exact opposite. In Rodolphe Töpffer's *Essay on Physiognomy*, he says that having identical noses does not make identical men.[51] Genetics is like that. Even having similar genes can allow us different personalities. Twin studies clearly show this.

Therefore, we now know that procrastination may be an evolutionary byproduct of impulsivity, and that the former indeed has a hereditable tendency. So if we end up wasting a lot of time in front of the TV, we have an excuse—perhaps our parents are to blame. After all, unlike a television, parents aren't replaceable—we may inherit their genetic scripts, but our actions become quills that reveal our individual handwriting.

Conclusion

Sui means "flowing" or "freeform," rather like water, in Japanese. Bodies are meant to be like that—flexible, supple, magnetic, and changing according to the seasons of our lives. After all, did we not originate from deep under the oceans?

Ultimately, everything boils down to the beautiful simplicity of movement. Evolution is analogous to life, and both are meant to be constantly on the move. After millions of years of evolution, we know this much is true: humans do what they do best when they are two legged. For many, this may mean tramping in mountains, fishing rivers, playing sports, farming, or simply walking. There have been sluggish people with sluggish genes who prevented us from ending up as fodder for wily predators. Pitted against this are genes that evolved to make us natural dancers and athletes. Everything happens for a reason. Our genetic memories depict our histories accurately; science merely follows the trail afterward.

Genetics tells us that genes are just as selfish as we are, even if evolution tries its darnedest not to make such things obvious. As humans became two legged, there were more reasons to move, and a larger brain evolved—full of brutishness, ego, and industrial zeal. But as more and more automation comes about, we seek to make things easier for humankind and move less, forgetting the reason for our brains becoming bigger in the first place. Therefore, unlike wild animals, our human populations have become fatter and fatter, and our muscles weaker and weaker. And, increasingly, it is obvious that all our visual and balance systems were optimized to make us modern humans upright and two legged. With the increasing use of cell phones, everyone you pass on the street seems hunched over their mobile devices, a sort of reverse evolution, the appearance of Homo mobilensis, a new species of man designed with the optimum body shape to work computers.

So, rather than being fun, movement has become a pain in the ass or something that must be forced upon us. Guess who modulated this slippery slope to slothfulness? Genes. All right, not particular genes, but several "gene associations," territories in genetic wastelands where disease-linked genes live in clusters. If you ask me, these are evolutionary excuses. What movement for movement's sake, like dance, has shown us is that we are still guinea pigs in an evolutionary lab. We could stop dancing, but then we'd end up having to depend on luck. No self-respecting species does things like that.

Reader Rx: Get Moving

Endurance exercises improve brain function, so pick something you like, start slow, and keep building endurance levels up. There are many different forms of endurance exercise and many involve leg movement, for example swimming, running, football, racket sports, aerobics, and dancing, so pick one that you like and make sure you vary it, so the procrastination gene does not set in. You don't have to worry about finding much time; averaging just thirty minutes a day has been shown to be beneficial. Remember, tango is especially beneficial for your brain, so look for lessons.

Key Points

1. The brain evolved for movement, not just to move muscles.
2. There are gene associations or evidence for "sluggish genes"; therefore, once we stop moving, it is harder to get going.
3. The major change from apes to man was the development of bipedalism (i.e., the ability to walk on two legs).

4. When exercises like yoga, Tai Chi, and tango were compared, even though all postural exercises help, ones that involve walking and impulsivity with a partner, like tango, have the greatest benefit in reducing dementia or improving Parkinson's disease.
5. The genetics of procrastination is related to the genetics of impulsivity.
6. Procrastination is also an evolutionary trait. The brain is slower to buy your plan, therefore forcing you to improve it.
7. Humans do what humans do best when they are two legged.
8. Movement is extremely important for both heart and brain fitness.

3

THE STRESS GENES: SABER-TOOTHED TIGERS AND SCAREDY-CATS

I am an old man now; I've had lots of trouble,
and most of it never happened.

—Thomas Dixon Jr.

Stress may be like math at school—a small mountain everyone has to master. At the Auckland University of Technology, where I'm an adjunct professor, I was discussing with a computer engineer how DNA is effectively our body's binary code. Computers store data in two-valued bits, binary digits that either have a value of 0 or 1. Our DNA stores data in four-valued base pairs, the sequences of which are called *genes*.

Like math, stress at a basic level is a necessary evil—useful for some, but for most a nuisance. Increasingly, research into evolutionary biology points to the genetic basis of stress.

Before a trip to Washington, DC, several years ago, I was invited to dinner by the US ambassador and asked for some travel advice regarding my destination. "DC has a lot of crime," I was told. "Stay at a hotel around Dupont Circle, and if you take the Metro, stick to the blue line; *avoid* the red line. Even areas around the White House can be unsafe at night." I made some mental notes.

Once I reached Washington, I enjoyed my time in DC. Per square mile, Dupont Circle must have the highest density of independent bookstores. Bookstores are a good hangout—even better when they have a brasserie attached as one I found did. I found Steven Pinker's *The Better Angels of Our Nature,* in which Pinker argues that even with terrorist threats and greater migration, we live in the safest of times. *He can't be right,* I thought. After all, even the American ambassador had advised me to avoid the Washington, DC, Metro's red line after dark. Pinker's book compares recorded homicide rates: in fourteenth-century London, the murder rate was about 100 per 100,000 people; now it is about 2 per 100,000. In late sixteenth-century Rome, it ran between 30 and 70 per 100,000 people; now it is closer to 1. In 2014, in Washington, DC, there were 15.9 murders for 100,000 people—still much safer than Rome or London in the fourteenth and sixteenth centuries.

If we live in the safest of times, why are we so anxious about danger? George Bernard Shaw once said, "There is always danger for those who are afraid."[1] As travelers, we worry about safety; as parents, we are anxious about our kids. My daughter is at university, and I worried about her when she told me about some of her "initiation" ceremonies. I couldn't sleep. I had forgotten that I also had been through university and survived my rites of passage.

Evolution is one big initiation for species. Nature is in the business of creating living things, and in the spirit of benevolent adventure, a few species are sacrificed; whole animal groups may be eliminated, only to be replaced by others. In prehistoric times, saber-toothed cats wreaked havoc on migrating humans. Now those beasts are gone; we are still here. That should be reason enough for us to feel positive, but as Elizabeth Kostova wrote in *The Historian*: "I have learned that, in fact, not everyone who reaches back into history can survive it. And it is not only reaching back that endangers us; sometimes history itself reaches inexorably forward for us with its shadowy claws."[2]

Saber-toothed tigers went extinct ten thousand to twelve thousand years ago, yet they put the fear of the devil into our very core.

"I'm not going to send you any more saber-toothed tigers," Nature says.

"But you're sure to send something else to trouble us," Man replies.

"Are you going soft on me?" Nature asks teasingly.

The truth is, we *are* going soft, but our muscular weakness belies our strength and cunning. However, the dangers our ancestors faced have already been embedded as stress genes in our archaic memory. What was once a necessity for survival has become a millstone around our skinny necks.

One way of assessing the risk of a particular process in biology is to look at what a particular function represents as a means of understanding eventualities. For example, when we are exposed to the sun, our skin tans. We know this is because melanin is an antioxidant, and therefore, tanning is a defense mechanism. It automatically follows that if sunburn were to create a lethal tumor, we would expect such a tumor to contain melanin, which is indeed what happens when people end up with a deadly melanoma after sunburn or sunbed use. Likewise, when we detect danger, we secrete stress-related chemicals. In short bursts, these chemicals are helpful. But when we begin to imagine danger everywhere, these chemicals wreak havoc on our bodies.

One of the hypocrisies of evolution is that it is supposed to be improving species, but stress, an evolutionary response, dominates our lives. Dealing with stress has become a game of frowns, with many battles, real and imagined. The stresses we deal with may not accurately reflect our real world, but diseases caused by stress become real—and stress genes are a source of genetic signals that are both traps and delusions. Life has ups and downs, and happiness does not have to be mandatory. What humans have to remember is stress is a real evolutionary learned response; it is our response to stress that is unreal. We simply have to cope better, for our own good. Paraphrasing Winnie-the-Pooh, we need to learn the art of just going along with life, listening to all the things (stressors) you can't hear, and not bothering.

The Evolution of Stress

I couldn't go to DC and not visit one of the Smithsonian museums. Anna Behrensmeyer, a paleontologist at the Smithsonian National Museum of Natural History, has a theory about early humans and saber-toothed tigers. She has concluded that this beast attacked and killed off an entire group of early humans: a grouping of hominids of the Australopithecus afarensis species—the tribe Lucy, the famous early "human" whose skeleton was found in Ethiopia in 1974, belonged to. Behrensmeyer studied these hominid skulls forensically at a spot in Ethiopia and found the hallmarks of a saber-toothed killer. Interestingly, Lucy got her name from the Beatles song "Lucy in the Sky with Diamonds," as this soundtrack was the favorite of that expedition team, led by Donald Johanson.[3]

This mass murder by a saber-toothed cat happened about 3.2 million years ago, yet saber-toothed tigers have retained their fearsome reputation down the centuries. These were big beasts, three hundred to six hundred pounds in weight and nearly four feet tall. The biological name of the American saber-toothed cat is *Smilodon fatalis*, which makes it sound like a smiling assassin. And it was. There are many theories about the reasons for the tusk-like teeth of these large cats, which were perhaps closer to modern lions than tigers. Some theories suggest that these tusks were used for climbing trees; others suggest that they helped with swimming. Some scientists have noted that as these large cats could disarticulate their lower jaws, it enabled them to use their tusks as mini-spears. Whatever the reason, these were among the most ferocious and awe-inspiring predators that have ever roamed the earth.

In 1794, William Blake wrote the poem "The Tyger" as part of his *Songs of Innocence and of Experience* collection. The poem reads:

> Tyger Tyger, burning bright,
> In the forests of the night;
> What immortal hand or eye,
> Could frame thy fearful symmetry?
> In what distant deeps or skies.
> Burnt the fire of thine eyes?
> On what wings dare he aspire?
> What the hand, dare seize the fire?
> And what shoulder, & what art,
> Could twist the sinews of thy heart?
> And when thy heart began to beat,
> What dread hand? & what dread feet?[4]

Mathematically, danger is often understood using the signal detection theory. We know that early humans lived when saber-toothed tigers roamed the world. Yet humans have outlived these animals. How did we manage that? This is where the sensory detection theory comes to the fore. We know that saber-toothed cats were felinely stealthy, and therefore, a human needed to know if a particular rustling noise was a saber-toothed cat or merely the wind.

I underwent this experience once, as a child, when my family sent me to Bombay (now Mumbai) to visit an uncle, and an office assistant was asked to give me a guided tour of the city and its surrounds. This young man didn't speak a word of English, and I didn't speak a word of Marathi, the local language. We were visiting some caves in the district, where there were rumored to be tigers. Every time the wind roared, it would send a chill up my spine and I would ask him if it was a tiger. He would respond reassuringly in his language and it stopped me from running away. To this day, I don't know if he was telling me whether it was the wind or if the tiger was too far away to worry about.

Ambient noise can be shown to fluctuate. Sometimes the wind may roar louder than a tiger; at other times, the tiger may cause the rustle as it seeks to rustle up a few humans for dinner; and there are times when the noise is merely in our minds. Each one of us has a signal detection threshold, a level of rustling that would make our brains accept the evidence that a tiger was present. Below our individual tiger thresholds, we will dismiss the sound as mere noise. Therefore, not only do we end up with some false alarms, but there are also often valid reasons for alarm—for example, in physically slow or lame animals, the tiger threshold may be lower to allow more time to escape. In simple terms, this means that animals respond to many perceived threats that aren't actual threats, but from an evolutionary perspective, it will likely pay off if even one of those scares is actually a predator and the animal gets to safety. This is nature and evolutionary biology at its finest. Borrowing from the principle of a smoke alarm, we pay a small cost up front to buy safety, or we suffer a fatal consequence. In other words, everything is designed to allow us to respond to danger when it is present. This is why the blind develop acute hearing and a heightened sense of touch.

Randolph Nesse first explained the signal detection theory in his book *Why We Get Sick: The New Science of Darwinian Medicine*.[5] Darwin himself noted that anxiety could be an adaptive response. A quote widely misattributed to Darwin is, "It is not the strongest of the species that survives, nor the most intelligent that survives. It is the one that is most adaptable to change." I've heard this quoted at both scientific and business conferences. I have read pretty much all of Darwin's writings, but I have never managed to find these words in any of his books. However, Darwin did say:

Instincts are not always absolutely perfect and are liable to mistakes; that no instinct has been produced for the exclusive good of other animals, but that each animal takes advantage of the instincts of others; that the canon in natural history of *natura non facit saltum* is applicable to instincts as well as to corporeal structure, and is plainly explicable on the foregoing views, but is otherwise inexplicable, all tend to corroborate the theory of natural selection.[6]

Anxiety is that kind of an instinct. Heightened anxiety evolved as a fight-or-flight response destined to save us from predators like saber-toothed cats. The overconfident, brave men probably charged out of their caves, spear in hand, challenging saber-toothed cats and ending up as feline fatalities. The anxious ones who imagined a saber-toothed cat at every corner survived to propagate the species. Therefore, the genes that controlled this stress response survived.

The feeling of anxiety is meant to be unpleasant, like the sound of an alarm, to ensure the affected creature is either forewarned or armed adequately. As Nesse said:

The strong, rapid heartbeat that accompanies panic anxiety brings extra nutrition and oxygen to muscles and speeds the removal of wastes. Muscle tension prepares for flight or physical defense. Shortness of breath induces rapid breathing, hyper-oxygenating the blood. Sweating cools the body in anticipation of flight. Greater production of blood glucose also helps bring more nutrition to the muscles. Secretion of adrenaline into the blood makes it clot faster, should injury occur. Blood circulation shifts from the digestive system to the muscles, leaving a cold, empty feeling in the pit of the stomach and a tense readiness in the muscles.[7]

More recently, researchers have found that there is a key difference between acute (short-term) stress and chronic (longer-term) stress; the former may indeed be beneficial. After all, the stress response was a learned response to a particular memory, and many of the chemicals secreted initially helped the animal cope and adapt. Studies on rats have shown that significant but brief stressful events caused stem cells in their brains to produce new brain cells and improve the rat's performance. These rats even lived longer. In contrast, when one was under stress for long periods, the chronic stress elevates glucocorticoid stress hormones levels. These steroid hormones suppress the production of new neurons in the hippocampus part of the brain, impairing memory and suppressing immune responses. Research also shows that acute stress triggers the release of a protein, fibroblast growth factor 2 (FGF2), by brain cells called astrocytes, but in chronic stress, FGF2 gets depleted and leads to depression. All this science simply confirms that too much of anything is bad for us—a rule that applies equally to Darwinism (stress), disease (pain), and dessert (sugar).

Worriers vs. Warriors

Researchers have also been looking at links between genes and the stress response. Can human beings be genetically classified into worriers and warriors? Before we get carried away by genomics, we need to go back to the old adage that our genes shape our environment, and our environment shapes our genes. If you grew up in an environment that made you a well-adjusted person, you may end up dealing with stress more easily. However, if you have a genetic predisposition toward depression, the loss of a loved one or a broken relationship could tip you over the edge more than it would affect someone with a different genetic personality.

First, to be stressful enough to activate these stress genes, it has to be something that drives us nuts with worry. NUTS is actually an acronym used to describe stressful situations: Novelty, Unpredictability, Threat to the ego, and/or diminished Sense of control.[8]

Second, twin and animal studies have shown that early maternal care affects a child's stress genes—nurture affects your nature. Rat babies, or pinkies, that were licked and shown more affection by their mothers produced less stress hormones and had better memories when compared to neglected siblings. When Michael Meaney, professor at McGill University Faculty of Medicine, studied rodents exposed to stressful and dangerous situations, his team found that rats raised by low-licking mothers responded to stress with larger increases in the stress hormone; this response is an adaptive response.[9] These rat pinkies became genetically programmed to interpret even ordinary environments as adverse and stressful, and therefore needed to mount larger stress responses to survive daily life. They became "stress rats" and everything seemed to worry them. Twin studies have also shown that someone who grew up without a loving mother ended up more neurotic.[10]

The way we deal with stress is honed in childhood. If you are a pack animal and constantly picked on, your body may sometimes seek to avoid the unpleasantness of the stress reaction and simply acquiesce. As we saw with the NUTS acronym, a constant sense of a lack of control—for example, if someone is in a controlling relationship—is often a stimulus for the stress response. This is called *learned helplessness* in evolutionary psychology and is the reason why stressful situations or depression may make people sleepy—while our bodies may avoid conflict by falling asleep, we're not really escaping anything. This kind of learned helplessness also explains why some kidnapped individuals have remained with their captors for years, especially those with a history of childhood abuse. This is a classic case of an adaptive response outliving its value. If you experience too many bad events, especially during your formative years, your stress response may become one of somnolent escapism or masterful inactivity.

For the first 1.5 billion years, all creatures had one cell. As they evolved into multicellular creatures, gradually certain cells began to perform specific functions. The next stage was the separation into somatic cells (cells that perform certain functions; precursors of organs) and sex cells (gametes, or reproductive cells, precursors of gonads). Many organs began as ambitious cells and then passed the evolutionary test to end up as permanent body parts in their own right. The primary purpose of multicellularity was communication. In the early stages, when life was simple, many creatures didn't have hearts or brains. Therefore, skin served as the sense organ of touch and, therefore, ended up our largest, omnipresent sensory organ.

In the early days, messages about external threats were sensed by the skin and not the brain, as creatures did not have a well-developed nervous system. The signals produced specific molecules that docked on the outside of cell walls, requested permission, and gained entry into the cell. To ensure that these signals didn't die out but kept getting passed on through the body of the creature, impatient proteins kept banging jungle drums, and these messages were coded by genetic signals.

In creatures that lack a nervous system, the skin warns the creature about threats. Later on, the nervous system took on this task, as it was full of neuronal wiring that made it efficient at transmitting signals to specific sense organs like the eyes, ears, and nose.

External signals can be good or bad, pleasant or unpleasant. Sensations are like news stories and possibly why we refer to some stories as "sensational." News, by nature, is both fickle and temporary. News stories don't last long, but they create a memory of things that have happened, and when such experiential messages become acute or chronic, they create evolutionary memoirs such as stress responses that endure still today.

But what of the difference between the sexes? Does that play a role in the stress response? In the early stages, all creatures were alike in a physical sense—both sex organs existed within the same crea-ture, and later species were separated into male and female. But this separation into male and female has led to major debates among evo-lutionary biologists. To begin with, sexual reproduction that involves two partners is far less efficient and more cumbersome than self-fertilization, so why did evolution allow this? The basic idea is that, if an organism reproduces asexually, then the genetic variation of its species as a whole will slowly grind to a halt—in other words, the primary purpose of sexual reproduction between two creatures was to ensure new genetic varieties.

In the animal kingdom, most males sleep all day (lions) or are killed during the honeymoon period (mosquitoes). It is generally the females that rear the young, while the males guard the territory. Therefore, it is only natural that they respond to stress differently. If stress is a fight-or-flight response, are males inherently fighters and women fretters?

When researchers looked at the difference in the genes associated with stress in males and females, they came across a gene called SRY that is found exclusively in men. Joohyung Lee, a neuroscientist at the Hudson Institute of Medical Research, and his colleague, Vincent Harley of Prince Henry's Institute, both affiliated to Monash University in Melbourne, suspected that the Y-chromosome gene SRY actually makes males more aggressive when faced with stress.[11] SRY plays a role in the heart, lungs, and brain. It's involved in the release of the neu-rotransmitter dopamine, which, as we noted in the previous chapter, is crucial for movement. SRY also shows up in the adrenal glands, which secrete adrenaline (epinephrine) and noradrenaline (norepineph-rine). These three chemicals are the main ones implicated in our stress response. SRY being a Y-chromosome-linked gene may explain why dopamine-related diseases like Parkinson's disease, autism, attention deficit or hyperactive disorders, and schizophrenia are more common in males. In the evolutionary scheme of things, men became warriors to fight off threats and women became worriers, as they had to nurture their offspring.

In recent times, advanced technologies combining radiology and genetics have increased our understanding of the genes that regulate the stress response. As we discussed in the previous chapter on movement, functional brain scans are increasingly useful in detecting activity in the brain. But how can we determine the actual genes that trigger things like anxiety? We've just hypothesized that stress and anxiety are evolutionary throwbacks to dangerous times. Recent advances in genetic science have led to the use of imaging genomics. Imaging genomics is a relatively new research technique that links functional gene variants and brain information processing—in other words, real-time scans are compared with genetic testing to see areas of the brain activated by specific genes.

Two chemicals that are implicated in stress have shown particular genetic linkages—serotonin (5-hydroxytryptamine or 5-HTT), a chemical known as a "mood stabilizer," and catechol-O-methyltransferase (COMT), an enzyme that breaks down dopamine, which I earlier called the "pleasure particle." Scans done on people in stressful situations particularly showed 5-HTT and COMT genes in the brain responding to stressful stimuli. The 5-HTT gene polymorphism (HTTLPR) is associated with anxiety in response to emotional situations, and a COMT Met158 gene allele leads to lower COMT activity and has also been associated with anxiety and adds to the effect of HTTLPR. People with Met158 genotypes are more sensitive to pain stress. In other words, they are more likely to have needle phobias or end up with problems with opiate addictions or pain syndromes.

Environment matters and modifies our genetic responses. In an article published in *Nature Neuroscience* and quoted in *Mammoth* magazine, German researchers studied stress in young rats by separating them from their mothers for three hours a day over ten days—what they felt was a relatively mild stressor.[12] What they found was astonishing. Even mild stress, once it became a regular occurrence (what we medically term *chronic*), ended up leaving a permanent epigenetic footprint—these rats developed variations in genes that code a protein involved in stress, namely vasopressin. Similarly, the genetic code for the NR3C1 gene is modified in the hippocampus of humans who were abused during childhood, and these people had a high risk of committing suicide.

Stress responses, as noted in many animal studies, some of which I've quoted, are not unique to humans. The genes that modulate anxiety are archaeological remains of lessons that were learned for species to survive and thrive in a dangerous and predatory world.

Stress in the Modern Age

Nassim Nicholas Taleb, the Lebanese American scholar who has written many books on randomness and probability, had this to say about modern lives in an essay titled "Stretch of the Imagination": "The difference between technology and slavery is that slaves are fully aware that they are not free."[13] Taleb is right. The advent of technology everywhere has meant no escape from friend or foe—and no freedom to go on solitary walkabouts to reconnect with our past as our ancestors did.

The problem of stress today lies within our imaginations. A dressing-down from a boss a century ago might have been settled with a punch. Today we're much less likely to be punched, but the anxiety is there regardless, as is fear of financial or other repercussions, despite the fact that these incidents on their own are not life threatening or physically harming. A visit to a doctor for a routine blood pressure check may induce a stress response at the thought of impending heart disease. In today's world, we see metaphorical saber-toothed tigers everywhere—in subways, schools, and sporting events—but instead of this fear subsiding when the tiger is gone, we continue to feel anxious, and the longer we feel stress, the more it affects our health. Anxiety genes that modulate our response to stress may have been protective and evolved as warning mechanisms, but now they have outlived their purpose.

In the animal kingdom, most animals live in groups or within packs, and it is not uncommon for males to compete for females. The males that lose the battle for dominance end up reconciling with their conqueror and accepting a subservient position, if only to ensure that they remain within the safety of the pack, thereby avoiding other predators. On the other hand, for beings used to a life of solitude, anything that shatters that idyll can be equally as threatening as the idea of being pushed out of a pack.

In Daniel Defoe's *Robinson Crusoe*, there is a scene where, after fifteen years of solitude, Crusoe finds a footprint on the sand of his supposedly uninhabited island. Until that moment, it had been only Crusoe and God on the island. Crusoe had complete control over the island. A footprint threatened that sense of control—a trigger for stress. Crusoe's mind began to play tricks on him:

> Terrify'd to the last degree, looking behind me at every two or three steps, mistaking every bush and tree, and fancying every stump at a distance to be a man; nor is it possible to describe how many various shapes my affrighted imagination represented things to me in, how many wild ideas were found every moment in my fancy, and what strange, unaccountable whimsies came into my thoughts by the way.[14]

Robinson Crusoe was written in 1719. In 1840, Charles Darwin read *Gulliver's Travels* and *Robinson Crusoe*.[15] Like the protagonist of Defoe's novel, Darwin was a reclusive figure, and for all his wisdom about evolutionary biology, he was not immune to anxiety disorders. Darwin suffered from weakness, hyperventilation, palpitations, and a poorly functioning immune system, leading many medical scholars to hypothesize that he'd been exposed to a virus or parasite possibly picked up during his voyages—diagnoses such as Chagas disease (caused by bloodsucking bugs endemic in South and Central America) or a post-viral myalgic encephalomyelitis (ME) have been suggested. No conventional treatments worked for Darwin, and he even tried water therapy at Dr. James Gully's Water Cure Establishment at Malvern.

Charles Darwin lost his mother when he was eight and remained a reclusive figure for most of his life. His father, Erasmus, was keen for him to study medicine. Even if Darwin himself wasn't, he was fearful of displeasing his father. At the University of Edinburgh, Darwin found the practice of surgery to be too brutal and ended up a scholar of natural history instead. A lack of a mother and living under a father who demanded high standards may have heightened Darwin's anxiety. His fear of failure led him to delay publication of his books for decades. He wrote to a fellow scientist, Robert Hooker:

> You ask about my book, & all that I can say is that I am ready to commit suicide: I thought it was decently written, but find so much wants rewriting . . . I begin to think that every one who publishes a book is a fool.[16]

In contrast to Darwin's reaction, while I was in the process of rewriting parts of this book during the final edits, I was thinking, *I thought it was decently written, but find so much wants rewriting. It's great that I am making these changes now, so it can be an even better book when we complete this process.*

Rejection and rewriting are staples in a writer's life. Stephen King, the prolific and prominent horror novelist, wrote about how his works were rejected over and over—more times than he could count: "By the time I was fourteen, the nail in my wall would no longer support the weight of the rejection slips impaled upon it. I replaced the nail with a spike and went on writing."[17]

King was able to look beyond the rejection. Darwin ended up getting his book finished, and it ended up being a major contribution to mankind, but he suffered a great degree of angst during the process and contemplated ending his life. On the other side of the coin, King also notes the importance of work enjoyment, stability, and managing stress as key reasons his career has been so successful and he's been so healthy:

> The combination of a healthy body and a stable relationship with a self-reliant woman who takes zero shit from me or anyone else has made the continuity of my working life possible. And I believe the converse is also true: that my writing and the pleasure I take in it has contributed to the stability of my health and my home life.[18]

Psychiatrists are now convinced that Darwin suffered from panic attacks and anxiety disorders, which would explain his secluded lifestyle as well as his difficulty in speaking before groups and socializing with colleagues.[19] Such social anxiety is, after all, a mechanism to avoid rejection or exclusion, and in Darwin's case, losing a mother so early may have been one of the causes. However, given that Darwin also was known to have a deficient immune system and was prone to illness, it is worth looking at the mechanisms of chronic anxiety disorders and stress and how they impact on our health.

The word *stress* derives from the Latin *stringere*, which means "to be drawn tight," literally high-strung. We can see where the term comes from and why Taleb's essay was titled "Stretch of the Imagination." Our imagination has the power to both set us free and enslave us.

Walter Bradford Cannon, who was a professor of physiology at Harvard Medical School, studied the body's stress response, including chronic stress, in detail. Cannon was fascinated by the work of the Frenchman Claude Bernard in describing homeostasis, the process by which the body maintains a steady state, which includes keeping the internal environment at a constant temperature, pressure, and pH, irrespective of the external environment.

Cannon wrote his book *Wisdom of the Body* in 1932 and described the flight-or-fight response as being the first response of an animal to stress.[20] He explained that the body secreted chemicals called catecholamines in response to threats. This early warning system is controlled subconsciously by the autonomous nervous system. This is an adaptive response by organisms for survival and improved the biological fitness of populations. Since the dawn of time, creatures have been exposed to threats to their existence that called for a flight-or-fight response for survival. Both fighting or fleeing carry the risk of injury and infection, and therefore, the body's response was to secrete chemicals that would help deal with wound repair, pain, and diseases.

The subconscious and adaptive manipulation of genes and hormones was an important part of evolutionary society. Pain and stress were important acute responses. We needed to sense danger; our limbs needed to know when they were injured to avoid further damage. But these evolved as acute, short-term responses. During my many travels, I've heard many sayings and one of my favorites is this: the mother of excess is not named Joy. And this appears to be a universal truism.

Cassandra Clare wrote in her fantasy novel *City of Lost Souls*, "Too much of anything could destroy you . . . too much darkness could kill, but too much light could blind."[21] Stress as a medical condition is a fantasy, a form of useful fiction, an old historical novel. The problem is when the stress or pain responses become excessive. When that happens, and the responses are long term, it causes deep psychological and physical illness; when pain becomes chronic, it ends up ruining lives. Both chronic stress and chronic pain are deeply debilitating conditions, and both can lead to suppression of the immune system due to the hormones involved. These responses are finely tuned alarms. But when the alarms keep going off, they create a deafening racket, and that sets up a vicious cycle—our attempts to dampen these alarms with bodily hormones, gene expression, and drugs are so frequently inadequate because, fundamentally, the more alarmed you get, the more chemicals you need, and these cause further alarms.

The three main chemicals that are lumped together as stress hormones are adrenaline (epinephrine), noradrenaline (norepinephrine), and cortisol.

Adrenaline is the fight-or-flight hormone, and therefore, its actions are not only immediate, but also designed to fight or flee—for example, it tenses your muscles and also gives you a surge of energy that can help you run away. Because its effect is immediate, it is used as a medication when someone has a serious allergic reaction. We secrete adrenaline when we swerve to avoid colliding with another car and can feel our hearts racing and chest pounding. As its name indicates, adrenaline is a product of our adrenal glands. Its effects are both immediate and short acting.

Noradrenaline is the arousal hormone and a cousin of adrenaline. This also is fast acting and makes us hyperalert and vigilant. This is what is secreted when we think we sense a burglar and it prepares us to flee. Given that the effects of both adrenaline and noradrenaline overlap, this hormone may seem redundant, but there are some differences. For a start, noradrenaline is secreted both by the adrenals and the brain. Further, it lasts a bit longer than adrenaline, and we may feel its effects for a couple of days. It also backs up adrenaline, in the event you have an adrenal gland problem and cannot produce adrenaline properly.

Cortisol is the real stress-or-survival hormone, and it's what many people think of first when they hear the word *steroid*. It helps us survive trauma or blood loss and is, therefore, useful to maintain blood pressure and also fluid balance. When the stress response persists or if someone is on steroid medication, they end up with fluid retention, high blood pressure, obesity, and a suppressed immune system.

The production of cortisol is a multistep process, taking minutes to be produced, so it is not immediate like adrenaline. First, the part of the brain called the amygdala serves as the threat-recognition monitor. The amygdala sends an intruder alert to the part of the brain called the hypothalamus, which releases corticotrophin-releasing hormone (CRH). CRH then tells the pituitary gland to release adrenocorti-cotrophic hormone (ACTH), which stimulates the adrenal glands to produce ACTH. Vasopressin, mentioned earlier, is also linked to CRH. Acute stress leads to rapid release of vasopressin from the hypothalamus along with CRH. Vasopressin is also an antidiuretic hormone and helps us conserve fluid during blood loss.

Cortisol reduces levels of serotonin (5-HT) and dopamine, which ends up causing mental health problems. Because of the complex brain-pituitary-adrenal feedback mechanism in the production of cortisol, if a person is under severe stress, ACTH may indeed be suppressed, leading to reduced cortisol levels. Researchers at Umeå University, Sweden, studied people suffering with bipolar diseases and depression after stressful situations and concluded that even lifelong conditions like bipolar disorders can be caused by stress.[22] What they found is, during the initial period, when stress hormone levels are high, the person becomes manic. And when the steroid levels drop due to hormonal feedback mechanisms, people end up depressed. This cycle keeps getting repeated in an evolutionary loop of hormonal ping-pong. There are many other chemicals involved in the stress response, such as GABA (gamma-aminobutyric acid), an amino acid that is a calming neurotransmitter. I've only listed the main players in this chapter.

But why has modern life become so stressful? Breakdown of the family unit has meant less nurturing from mothers or periods of maternal absence. Further, increasing inequality and poverty means that people lower on the socioeconomic scale are more exposed to abusive behavior and poor diets full of chemicals. Substance abuse is rife. Technological advances and neoliberalism have led to greater unemployment, more sedentary lives, and feelings of lack of control or constant surveillance. There is also an obesity epidemic—human evolution has almost become survival of the fattest. High-calorie and high-sugar diets are a major problem, because when we eat high-sugar diets, they trick the brain into thinking we have not eaten enough— cells that secrete leptin, the "fullness hormone" are dulled; leptin is related to dopamine, which, in turn, is affected by both stress and lack of movement, as we noted in the previous chapter. Remember the stress hormones adrenaline and noradrenaline? Well, dopamine is a precursor chemical of both of those hormones and also has some receptors in the adrenal glands. Dopamine is related to pleasure-inducing activities, and reduced leptin, in turn, causes depression and anxiety.

Recently, researchers decided to study the link between our cafeteria diets (sodas and processed foods), obesity, and stress levels. They put female rats on cafeteria diets and fed them things like Coke, cookies, and potato chips—naturally the rodents became overweight.[23] The researchers concluded, "Obese and stressed female rats presented a higher anxiety index and predictive behavior for depression."

In short, there is a plethora of reasons why modern humans have as high or higher stress than ever before, and the effects of this chronic stress are never good. That's why we must keep our chins up, as the saying goes, and not take our troubles to bed.

Speaking of chins, I've always found them fascinating, in an anatomical sense. As a medical doctor and an animal biologist that is sometimes called to operate upon animals, I've often noted that humans are the only creatures with chins. But having a strong chin, psychologically rather than anatomically speaking, may be an even greater advantage, especially as our lives become busier and more controlled.

The Stressed Heart

In *Anne Grey*, an 1834 novel by Harriet Grove, one of the characters dies of a broken heart after losing a child: "Mrs. Daventry died of a broken heart. It was really of a broken heart, although Mr. Daventry did assure himself and his friends that this could not have been the case."[24]

Can one die of a stress-induced heart attack when her cholesterol and arteries are normal? In 1990, Professor Hikaru Sato and his cardiologist colleagues in Tokyo studied patients suffering heart attacks.[25] They noted that while these patients did not have coronary disease, they had been under intense stress that was overwhelming. When the hearts were examined, Sato felt that the apex of the left ventricle had ballooned out, and this chamber of the heart looked like a Japanese fisherman's octopus pot, the *tako-tsubo*, which is where the stress-induced syndrome that causes heart-muscle damage derived its name: Takotsubo cardiomyopathy.

In Western medicine, we call this *broken-heart syndrome*—more than 90 percent of reported cases are in women with normal coronary arteries, aged fifty-eight to seventy-five, who experienced chest pain and shortness of breath after severe stress (either emotional or physical). Stressful events that triggered such responses were varied, from car accidents to loss of a pet or spouse.

A surge of catecholamines, the hormones we discussed earlier, seems to cause muscle tensions that lead to rupture of the heart. Well-known bodily catecholamines are adrenaline and dopamine, neurotransmitters that Nesse noted as part of an animal's response to stress. Therefore, people who are under severe emotional stress when faced with traumatic situations are more prone to cardiac events.

Stress hormones affect the heart both acutely and chronically. As we noted earlier, the stress response causes an increased heart rate, muscle tension, and sweating. This is the acute phase of severe stress and may cause broken-heart syndrome. However, long-term or chronic stress is also equally damaging to the heart due to the persistent secretion of chemicals that raise blood pressure and heart rate. In 2007, a paper called "Chronic Stress and the Heart" in the *Journal of the American Medical Association* explained:

> Chronic stress has been shown to increase the heart rate and blood pressure, making the heart work harder to produce the blood flow needed for bodily functions. Long-term elevations in blood pressure (this can also be seen with essential hypertension, i.e. high blood pressure not related to stress) are harmful and can lead to myocardial infarction (heart attack), heart failure, abnormal heart rhythms, and stroke.[26]

Charles Dickens wrote in *Barnaby Rudge*, "There are strings in the human heart that had better not be vibrated."[27] He may well have been talking about the stress response triggers. Stress shocks the cardiac system, and our pre-eminent organ finds itself stunned by chemicals, leading to an aberrant anatomy and fugitive physiology that does not belong to a healthy heart.

Glycation—Precursor to Diabetes and Advanced Aging

There is a Chinese proverb that says that you can't expect both ends of a sugarcane to be as sweet. Indeed, sugar is a sweet-tasting hazard. While glucose is essential for cells, this can be produced from other dietary sources, so sugar is not essential in our diets. In olden days, the only way to add sugar was to use honey. Today, with our processed high-sugar foods, sickening sweetness is everywhere. If there is too much sugar in the body, protein molecules can cross-link with sugar molecules. The resultant "sugar proteins" are called *advanced glycation end products* (AGEs). Given that I also run a skin and cosmetics research lab, I originally became interested in AGEs because they make us age faster.

But recent research shows that stress also induces glycation. Glycation generates various compounds mediated by the human Receptors of AGE (RAGE) gene that is found on chromosome 6. We've known glycation is caused by too much sugar over a long time—after all, glycated hemoglobin (HbA1c) is used to measure and monitor diabetes. Can emotional stress worsen glycation and, therefore, also result in higher glycated hemoglobin, which is implicated in diabetes?

A team of medical researchers in Germany studied blood sugar levels in a group of medical students during examinations and concluded, "Longer examination periods significantly increased HbA1c percentage in healthy medical students; several months after the stressful examinations, the values were significantly lower."[28] These findings are especially significant, as this happened in healthy, nondiabetic individuals, yet psychological stress increased glycation, and therefore prolonged stress can increase your risk of diabetes.

Glycation, even when due to stress as opposed to diet, is also at play in how quickly we appear to age. In our world, where vanity is fair and youthful beauty is everything, increased research is now focused on AGEs. Glycation in skin reduces elasticity and increases wrinkles, as AGEs bind to collagen protein. Therefore, in people with higher sugar intake, diabetes, or high stress, the skin elasticity curve shifts downward, confirming that glycation stress is a major factor in the reduction of skin elasticity. Therefore, reducing sugar intake and stress and increasing muscular exercise helps one look younger. Muscle load or weight training is particularly important as well, as more than 70 percent of blood glucose is consumed in skeletal muscle and the more muscle one maintains, the less insulin resistance—if tissue becomes less resistant to insulin, its cells can break down sugar better using insulin. Meanwhile, from pharmaceutical companies to universities, AGE research seems to be the rage.

So stress can increase glycation, putting us at risk for diabetes and making us age faster. With the interest in glycation and its effect on aging came investigations into which diets could make one appear younger by reducing glycation. I'm constantly asked about diet and aging and if there are specific "skin foods." Reducing sugar intake is a must; vitamin C and E and things like green tea, blueberries, tropical ginger, and brazil nuts (due to high selenium levels) have all been shown to reduce glycation, and thereby AGE.

The Skin Carries the Stress

George Orwell once said, "At age fifty, everyone gets the face they deserve."[29] Skin would agree with that. As we approach fifty, we are leaving behind years where the impact of our dermal history may not be apparent to everyone—and then our exterior demonstrates that skin is essentially a mural of our lifestyle. In essence, the younger your skin looks, the fitter your bodily systems are. Emotional stress affects the overall picture.

Does age make things seem stressful, or is it stress that ages you? Joachim Fuchsberger, a German author, wrote the book *Altwerden ist nichts für Feiglinge*, which means "Age is not meant for cowards."[30] At what age do things start going downhill?

In general, larger animals seem to have slower metabolic rates and longer lifespans. Max Kleiber, a Swiss agricultural biologist from Zurich, did pioneering work in the 1930s comparing the metabolic rates of different animals. Kleiber's law, named after him, which is sometimes called the *mouse to elephant curve*, states that a creature's basal metabolic rate is proportional to three-quarters the power of an animal's mass: $R \propto M^{3/4}$.

But is it size or metabolic rate that really matters? Tortoises are smaller than elephants but have very slow metabolisms; some live for 150 years. Therefore, some scientists like Professor Thomas Kiørboe of the Centre for Ocean Life at the National Institute for Aquatic Resources, based at the Technical University of Denmark, feel that Kleiber's law may be too simplistic and cannot be applied across all species.[31]

A better way to understand aging is via the concept that every species has a maximum energy expenditure. All metabolic processes in the body generate free radicals, and these reactive oxygen species (ROS) are thought to be the major driving force behind the aging process. The first person to realize that even oxygen can be harmful in excess was the French nobleman and chemist Antoine Lavoisier, a man credited with discovering both oxygen and hydrogen. Lavoisier found that guinea pigs died under the influence of pure oxygen and mentioned that oxygen could be poisonous under certain circumstances.[32]

The more emotional or physical stress, the faster one's metabolism is due to secretions of catecholamines, and the more free radicals are produced. Therefore, not only does stress make you feel ill, as it did for Darwin, but it also makes you look older. I've often been asked about skin and stress. In my book *Dermocracy: By Brown Skin, For Brown Skin*, I go into detail about the negative effects of the stress response and skin. Dr. Howard Murad, a noted dermatologist who has written a book, *Conquering Cultural Stress: The Ultimate Guide to Anti-Aging and Happiness*, also talks about reducing stress to improve skin: "Don't focus on the minutiae in life. When you come to a wall in the road, life is telling you to make a turn. Go for it."[33] Managing stress becomes extremely important if you want to look younger.

As part of my research into skincare and cosmetics, I have a scanner that uses fluorescence spectroscopy to analyze skin. I can map out wrinkles present and emerging wrinkles. One of the things that I noted as I was analyzing wrinkles is that science has shown that the more wrinkles patients have on their cheeks, near their ears, the more likely they have heart disease—or the higher their risk of heart disease would be. This should have been obvious, given what I knew about glycation and how it affects aging, diabetes, and heart disease, but I hadn't thought of this fact much.

The lifespan of a keratinocyte, which is the predominant cell type in the epidermis, the skin's outer layer, is about a week, which means that the epidermal (outer) layers of skin reflect different life stages of keratinocytes as well as the environment we are living in, both internal (diet) and external (pollution). Think about this for a minute—if a keratinocyte starts in the deep, interior layers of the skin and lives for one week, gradually making its way to the outer surface of the skin during that week, then the skin's outer layer is a mirror of what is going on weekly inside our bodies.

Anne Tybjærg-Hansen, a clinical professor at Copenhagen University and a chief physician at the Department of Clinical Biochemistry at the Copenhagen University Hospital, studied this very phenomenon and said in 2012, "Our findings show that earlobe creases, cholesterol deposits on the eyelids, bald spots, and a receding hairline reflect the body's biological age and not just the chronological age."[34] This study started as early as in 1976 as part of the comprehensive Copenhagen General Population Study and was thirty-five years in the making. The study was interesting on two fronts. On one hand, it studied outer signs of chronological aging and what these revealed about our biological aging. Cholesterol deposits on the eyelids, earlobe creases, bald spots, and receding hairlines could indicate that the body's biological age was older than its actual chronological age. Wrinkles, on the other hand, reveal nothing about the body's biological age, but as research shows, wrinkles in certain locations on the face indicate an increased risk of developing heart disease.

In another of my books, *Skin, A Biography*, I go into detail about how nature and evolution have a way of being *satisficed*. The word was first used by Herbert A. Simon. In 1956, Simon came up with a portmanteau combining *satisfy* and *suffice*: satisfice. Another portmanteau is the word *redox*, which is a portmanteau of *reduction* and *oxidation*, more commonly known as oxidation reduction. When cells come under stress, such as due to UV rays causing sunburns, free radicals are generated. Free radical reactions are also generated by redox reactions when microorganisms attack the body. These radicals occur as part of a defense mechanism to ensure cell stability (a process termed *homeostasis*) by killing microorganisms using a process where an electron detaches from a molecule and then reattaches almost instantaneously. Free radicals are a part of redox molecules and can become harmful to the human body if they do not reattach to the redox molecule or an antioxidant. Unhitched free radicals can spur the mutation of cells they encounter and are, therefore, implicated in cancers.

A good way to understand free radicals and antioxidants is within the context of the stress response. As we discussed earlier, when human beings or animals get stressed, we secrete stress chemicals such as adrenaline, noradrenaline, and cortisol. When individual cells get stressed, they produce these ROS, or free radicals. This is a stress response on a microscopic scale—a stress response that survived from primitive creatures and microscopic microbes. For example, oxidative stress usually stops cells from dividing, thereby preventing any damaged genes from being transferred further. Without these free radicals, we'd die of infections. However, they can be produced in excess during stress—whether oxidative stress or anxiety-related conditions—and, in turn, can induce aging or illness.

From a biological point of view, aging can be understood simply as an accumulation of damage—progressive damage to individual cells, local tissues, and organs that ultimately leads to some organs failing and inevitable death. Being our largest organ, an envelope and a rampart against raging environmental factors, makes skin vulnerable to both external and internal damage. For example, toxins we ingest and emotional stress may cause cellular damage that the skin may end up reflecting, while getting weather-beaten or sunburned causes fine wrinkles, loss of elasticity, and reduced epidermal and dermal thickness. In today's world, the skin serves as the stress response's litmus paper.

Mood and Worry

We know that someone is feeling anxious or depressed just by looking at them. An aware person also knows this when they look in a mirror. However, there are subtle differences between stress, anxiety, and fear. If you are crossing the road and nearly get hit by a car, the initial response you feel is fear. The racing heart, sweating, and muscle tension that result are part of your stress response (which, in the short term, is, as we discussed earlier, normal). If you went back to that street a few days later and, with no car visible, relived the moment in your mind by developing the symptoms of stress, that is anxiety. Anxiety is essentially imagined fear.

It is worth looking at the role of serotonin (5-HT), which is a brain chemical that is biochemically derived from tryptophan, in the fear response—a trait that carried over from our saber-toothed cat days. Fear is usually a conditioned reflex. Initially, there is a neutral conditional stimulus, for example, the rustling of leaves; however, when this is paired with a dangerous end result, like the shock of seeing a mate dragged away by a saber-toothed beast, the original conditional stimulus itself arouses fear. If an animal had repeated conditional stimuli in the absence of danger, a repeated cry-wolf scenario, then the fear response would die down. After saber-toothed animals became extinct, humans may have still imagined these beasts for some time when they heard rustling leaves or soft footfalls.

Serotonin is very much involved in fear learning and fear extinction, and these are mediated by the interactions of various parts of the brain—mainly the amygdala, the hippocampus, and the bed nucleus of the stria terminalis. The latter contributes to unpredictable stress and anxiety.

What research has confirmed is that serotonin levels are increased in the amygdala in both cued and context-based fear conditioning, and there is a difference between imminent fear response and a sustained fear: if a person cannot reconcile these two, anxiety manifests itself. Scientists have now identified genes that regulate serotonin and that influence this fear conditioning. In humans, the short (s) allele, one of the genetic twins at the serotonin promoter region, is associated with abnormal anxiety—humans with two copies of these not only show increased fear responses, but they also exhibit a stronger startle response when surprised by sudden noise or other stimulus.

When it comes to the brain, there are three neurotransmitters: dopamine, serotonin, and noradrenaline. Dopamine is primarily concerned with movement and pleasure; serotonin and noradrenaline are primarily involved with mental behavior, be it fear or mood.[35]

The locus ceruleus (LC) of the brain is the primary source of noradrenaline, the stress chemical in the brain, and is considered a primitive part of the brain, which isn't surprising since the stress response is an ancient pathway. These LC neurons contain melanin (more on melanin in chapter 5) and, therefore, are dark in color. The LC not only dilates your pupils but also optimizes your attention and ability to assess the environment around you. When the LC is not working in the brain due to disease or destruction, you do not have an accelerated heart rate and the like when exposed to stress. As I mentioned, pain and stress are evolutionary warning systems, and it's only when they become long term that they are a problem. The LC also increases its firing in chronic pain situations, where inflammatory pain predominates.[36]

Let's try and simplify the brain anatomy and the stress response from an anatomical perspective. Previously, I was talking about the neurochemicals that are involved, not which regions of the brains were the culprits. The stress response anatomically works like this:

you sense a threat because you hear some rustling in the bushes. This triggers your amygdala, your early warning system; if the threat seems real to you, the amygdala communicates with the LC, and this secretes chemicals to help you prepare to fight or flee. The pathway is illustrated in my diagram below:

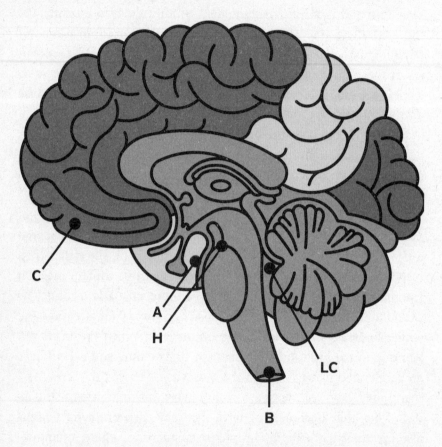

LC: Locus ceruleus (produces noradrenaline, the stress chemical)
H: Hippocampus (the part of the brain associated with learning and emotion)
A: Amygdala, your early warning system (the part that senses the "rustle in the bushes")

C: Cortex, the folded gray matter of the brain—mindfulness and meditation increase gray matter density

B: Brain stem: Controls breathing, blood pressure, heart rate as well as communicates messages from the brain to the rest of the body

All right, we think, *we've got some fancy anatomical warning systems in the brain to protect us, but what good are these monitoring structures without emotions to test them periodically and keep our alarms in working order?* Jean François Fernel, the French physician, once wrote: "Anatomy is to physiology as geography is to history; it describes the theatre of events."[37]

Is anxiety merely a manifestation of our scaredy-cat gene? How can we deal with anxiety or depression when it manifests? While therapy may be indicated for some, most of us need to accept that fluctuation in moods and fear are normal and ancient animal responses.

René Descartes, the seventeenth-century French philosopher, put forth the philosophical proposition, "I think, therefore I am."[38] With regard to stress, a corollary would be, "we stress, therefore we cope." If an entity such as the stress response exists, and it manifests at a cellular and biochemical level, as we've just covered, there must automatically be coping mechanisms. Indeed, studies now confirm that there is a brain circuit of serotonin-based neurons that connect the brain's cortex and amygdala through serotonin and glutamate receptors.

Foods such as coffee or tea have a fifth taste (other than sweet, sour, salty, and bitter) called *umami* that is related to receptors for the amino acid glutamate. Even breast milk contains umami flavor, and given that we've seen how the stress response relates to early maternal nurturing, these umami taste sensors are linked to our stress response genes. While glutamate is responsible for this umami taste, research shows that the interplay between glutamate and serotonin modulates our anxiety-related behavior.[39]

The link between taste receptors and fear response is interesting—and is perhaps why animals can smell or taste fear. We now know that the concentration required for a taste to be perceived, for a person to detect whether a food is sweet or bitter, varies according to levels of—guess what—serotonin. However, the same does not hold true for salty, sour, and umami. At the Umami Symposium at the European Sensory Network Seminar in Porto, Portugal, Dr. Lucy Donaldson, lecturer in physiology at the University of Bristol, UK, noted the link between the umami taste and anxiety: "If we plot the general anxiety levels against the umami threshold, what we find is that there is an inverse relationship . . . it's the opposite of the other tastes."[40] In other words, the more one can taste umami flavors—foods such as coffee, tea, soy sauce, shiitake mushrooms, Parmesan cheese, and so on—the more anxious the personality.

The link between serotonin and its mediation of our stress/anxiety responses is well-documented. But a problem arises when the same rule is applied for depression, something that pharmaceutical drug companies have done with great vigor. The issue with this is that, fundamentally, something that was a biochemical mechanism to deal with stress ended up becoming industrialized in the form of medications called *selective serotonin reuptake inhibitors*, or SSRIs. Drugs that supposedly restore serotonin levels have become all too common. While, by definition, an SSRI should increase serotonin levels by inhibiting reuptake, or reabsorption, of serotonin, the problem is no one really knows if they raise or lower levels, or if such changes are simply cyclical. In April 2015, *TIME Magazine* ran an article titled "Is the Link Between Depression and Serotonin a Myth?" wherein the magazine quotes Dr. David Healy, author of *Let Them Eat Prozac*, who says:

Drug companies marketed SSRIs for depression, even though they were weaker than older tricyclic antidepressants, and sold the idea that depression was the deeper illness behind the superficial manifestations of anxiety... the approach was an astonishing success, central to which was the notion that SSRIs restored serotonin levels to normal, a notion that later transmuted into the idea that they remedied a chemical imbalance.[41]

As Jonathan Leo and Jeffrey Lacasse wrote in an essay in the influential *PLoS Medicine* journal titled "A Disconnect between the Advertisements and the Scientific Literature," when researchers increased serotonin levels, they did not find they were able to alleviate depression.[42] Conversely, a lowering of brain serotonin also did not cause depression. Yet drugs that may help anxiety or obsessive behavior are increasingly peddled to people with depression and low mood in society's pursuit of happiness. It isn't that some of these psychiatric drugs don't work for depression; it is merely that the science is lacking when these drugs are used for depression, especially mild depression. Prozac, the best-known and best-marketed antidepressant, is one of the largest-selling drugs of all time. Originally developed as an anti-obesity drug, the pharmaceutical company decided on its use for treating depression, extending the anxiety-response analogy that does not stack up, in my view, when applied to depression. In its heyday, Prozac broke billion-dollar sales year after year. Later, similar drugs like sertraline (Zoloft) became the sixth bestselling medication in the United States in 2004, with over $3 billion in sales.

A friend who went to medical school with me is now a medical director of global medical and scientific affairs for a major pharmaceutical company and lives in Belgium. When we met for lunch in London during my last trip to the UK, I mentioned my concerns about the lack of science in psychiatry, especially depression and SSRIs. She agreed, saying that many drug companies have realized this and, therefore, don't invest a lot in research in mood-altering drugs; they simply recycle old medications by resurrecting them for new uses.

Serotonin is an interesting chemical that can also explain the "winter blues." We all know plants respond to light by producing chlorophyll. In actual fact, tryptophan, a precursor of serotonin, also captures light and is present in chlorophyll. This serotonin is involved in root growth and leaf motility, as well as being a potent antioxidant. However, animals lack chlorophyll, and we get our tryptophan and, therefore, serotonin from foods like almonds, brown rice, chocolate, dairy, and shellfish. That's why oysters and chocolates have a reputation as aphrodisiacs. Both contain chemical components that stimulate serotonin production. What would Thanksgiving be without turkey, another tryptophan-rich food? Also, the less sun, the less melanin, and the less serotonin, which is why people tend to feel low or depressed in winter and why sunny days make us feel happier.

The point is high serotonin does make us feel brighter and low serotonin makes us feel low, but clinical depression, the chronic state of low mood, cannot be as easily explained. Lowering serotonin does not automatically make one depressed, and this is where the science behind antidepressants becomes dodgy. Just because a drug lacks scientific evidence is not to say that it can't work, as we noted earlier, but perhaps if we acknowledge this, the pills would be a lot lighter on the pocket.

Tryptophan has also been implicated in various mood changes. When healthy volunteers had their diets supplemented with tryptophan for a fortnight, they recognized happy expressions in other people and disregarded disgusted faces.[43] Therefore, they generally felt more positive, and that's why many people feel chocolate is a comfort food. Interestingly, tryptophan did not alter perception of fear, however, because this was a trait needed for survival and not comfort.

Stress and Cancer

We've discussed the stress reaction and how it is evolutionarily entwined with our fear response. As noted, stress can cause heart disease, raise sugar levels, make your skin age faster, and affect your brain chemicals, leading to anxiety and depression. But can stress induce cancer? There has been no clear-cut scientific evidence to back this claim, and I myself hadn't really considered it, even if it seemed plausible, until I met Robert and Raewyn, who'd been married for 75 years.

There was a time when a tree grew right where the walls of my medical practice were built. It was a large oak tree with roots that had to make way for layers of concrete, wooden frames, and glass. Then the city council decided to widen the road and add traffic signals. Now, where it once stood is a square building with three consulting rooms and two nurses, and a shingle makes the only sign, but the tree keeps growing even though you can't see it anymore.

Today Robert has made his usual preparation. He has bought twenty-four empty bottles, a home-brew kit, and sprigs of herbs. These are all his favorite ingredients for his one-man beer fest. This happens every May, when winter is close to setting in in the Southern Hemisphere. Stay home and make his own spiced beer—that's what he likes to do. He used to like to get drunk at the veterans' bar, but all his army veteran friends are no more. The good thing about drinking alone is that you can do what you like. But he's actually not alone. He has a lovely wife, Raewyn. Except she can't drink anymore, as the doctor says it overloads her heart. But no one tells you off for getting drunk on home brew when you are at home listening to the radio.

He brings me a couple of bottles of his brew as a gift. I accept gratefully. I don't tell him that I never drink beer home-brewed by incontinent men. Certain times in life, you receive gifts that you know you are privileged to receive even if you don't like or need them. And you just take them with gratitude for the kindness of thought.

Raewyn and Robert are in their nineties and have hardly spent time apart in their decades of marriage, if you don't count the war years. Robert is thin and his hair has receded to the point where you can see all the precancerous growths on his head sticking out like barnacles. His baldness makes it easy for me to treat the skin cancers, and today I scrape and cut out several. "That's what being imprisoned in Singapore does to you," he tells everyone who is willing to listen. Raewyn, you can tell, used to be young and pretty once, and her weary eyes still have an arresting purple hue. But her heart is twice as large as it should be and her legs are filled with fluid that makes her socks soggy. Robert doesn't mind that. He always knew she had a large heart, he says. Heart failure, the doctor has called it. Failing heart or not, Raewyn insists on cooking a roast every Wednesday. She makes little slits in the meat to press garlic and pepper into. When there is garlic left over, she spreads it on the meat. There is no point in throwing anything away. Besides, garlic is good for the heart.

Raewyn and Robert are in my consulting room.

They are thinking of going to a rest home, they say.

"And you have decided that it would be best?"

"I'm not sure," Robert says. "I was thinking if something happened to me and Raewyn was alone, with her poor health, she wouldn't be able to manage."

"What about your kids?"

Their daughter is in Rotorua and is of the opinion that it is better for them sell and go to the rest home, they tell me.

"All right, if that's what you want, I'll get a social worker to show you around the rest homes," I say. "And, if you finally decide to take the plunge, I can arrange for a geriatrician assessment."

"That's good. Are we allowed to see if we like a rest home . . . as a sort of trial?"

"Of course you can."

"And if we are in a rest home . . . can I still have you as my skin doctor?"

"Of course."

Raewyn had accepted Robert's argument that if something should happen to him, she'd need to be looked after in a rest home. She didn't like rest homes but saw no reason to fuss. One does not fuss over things like that after so many years together. The social worker took them around to a few rest homes, but to Raewyn, the places lacked a soul. Sure, they were full of aging buildings and nurses who meant well, but something was lacking. You could put up flowery wallpaper, use fresh bed linens, and set out flowers, but she would still call them houses and not homes. The first one they visited had a garden where most of the plants looked crushed, as if their spirits had been trampled.

In the end, they decide to try a rest home out for a few weeks. The strange thing about rest homes is that time passes differently there than when you are at home. Sometimes Raewyn wondered if the time passed at all. She told Robert that they really should go home, and he agreed. He agreed even though he had reservations. He kept these to himself, so she wouldn't see his doubts. They'd been there only a fortnight. Everything takes time. *Time may stand still there, but their bodies continued to age*, Robert thought. We have got to go back home, he said. The look of elation in Raewyn's eyes told him that the decision was the right one. Let's check out, they decided, pretending they had honeymooned in a hotel for a week.

They went back home, except nothing was like they left it. A rough deck was added, a few children were playing on a trampoline. It was as if the house had gone on a trial of its own, taking on a new family. The girl on the trampoline looked strangely at the old couple and called out for her father. The lawyer showed them a sheet of paper. "Your daughter sold your house," the lawyer said.

"No way," Robert replied. "We were only going to the rest home for a trial. She can't do that!"

"I'm sorry, but she can," the lawyer said. "Remember, you signed a power of attorney?"

The trial was over. Let's go back to the rest home, they decided. It was time to retire and let living nightmares eat away at the spirits.

"You've decided to come back?" the doctor asked.

"Yes." Even in their distress, they couldn't betray their daughter—what would people think of her if they knew the truth?

A few assessments later, the home had bad news for them. "We can't house you together. Raewyn has dementia and is a safety risk. She will be housed in a secure wing. You, Robert, will get a nice room here, overlooking the park."

Robert could not make sense of what the doctor was saying. Can't be housed together? They'd been housed together for seventy-five years, right from when she stole his heart behind the changing sheds at the rugby club. They may have been far south of youth, but separation had never crossed their minds.

They would have to manage. Like they always had done.

The doctor at the rest home smiled the smile of an executioner. "If you need anything, just ask," he said.

They would have to live out the ends of their lives in solitude except for brief meetings during visiting hours. The food was passable. The doors creaked and seemed to say, "Everyone enters here once. No one leaves alive."

They entered at their own risk.

A few months later, I had a call from the rest home. Would I come and see Robert? He was unwell and couldn't make it to my clinic. The rest home had a GP but did not have a skin specialist. When I went to see him, he had a large lymph node mass on his neck and had developed several cutaneous lumps. Of course, he had sun-damaged skin and a high risk of skin cancer. But I had seen him barely two months earlier and examined him from head to toe. These lumps had not been present.

Two months later, he was gone, claimed by lymphoma. "They've taken Robert away from me," she said. Those were Raewyn's last words.

Medicine produces some cringeworthy moments that get etched onto your brain—errors you've made while prescribing drugs, postoperative complications, or hateful comments made by competing doctors with elaborate senses of self-importance or envy. I've coped with all of them. But to this day, my mind goes back to an old man who was robbed by his daughter, separated from his soul mate, and then became riddled with metastatic cancer. I can hear my inner voice contradicting published medical literature: *I know it was the daily stress that caused this.*

Can emotional stress cause serious diseases? This was the question Dr. Thomas Holmes asked himself in Seattle in the 1950s. Holmes conducted a series of experiments to study people who had suffered divorce, bereavement, or loss of a job. While Holmes's methods lacked the detail of modern biostatisticians, he reported that persons who had experienced stressful situations, such as divorce, death of a spouse, or loss of a job, were more likely to develop tuberculosis and less likely to recover from it.[44] Attempting to link diseases of the body with the mind did not go down very well with his medical peers. A commentator described his work as "complete baloney,"[45] yet many doctors who are interested in mind-body medicine see him as a pioneer. Holmes essentially challenged tuberculosis as a straightforward infection. While infection with the bacillus was necessary, he felt that psychological and social factors impacted the development of the disease.

Holmes's theories were not that far-fetched. According to the World Health Organization (WHO) and the Centers for Disease Control (CDC), a third of mankind, over two billion people, are infected with tuberculosis, yet in 2011 only 8.7 million people fell ill with TB and 1.4 million died from it.[46] Given that stress levels affect immunity and that TB is strongly linked to deficient cell-mediated immunity, Holmes wondered if low stress meant stronger immune systems. That was the kind of logic Holmes applied to his clinical studies; however, as there are many factors, like overcrowding and malnutrition, that increase the stress response and risk of TB, people discredited his research.

In some ways, it was a pity that Holmes chose TB. Given that the mycobacterium is well studied and the mechanism of infection is well-known, it led many in the mainstream medical establishment to criticize his work and think of it as pseudoscience. He realized this later on. But Holmes's basic supposition was correct—stress reduces immune responses and can cause serious illness.

But what about cancer?

Until recently, there was not much evidence regarding cancer and psychological stress as a causative agent. However, studies have shown that stress can alter a potentially important defense mechanism against malignant diseases; stress can not only alter natural killer (NK) cell activity, but can also negatively affect the ability of NK cells to respond and be effective in the killing of appropriate tumor-infected or virally infected cells.[47]

Studies have shown an association between stressful life events and higher incidences of cancer of the lungs, breasts, and colons. Ronald Glaser, physician and director of the Institute for Behavioral Medicine Research at Columbus, Ohio, has now collated an impressive collection of research articles on the effects of stress on cancer, showing that stress causes immune suppression, affects DNA repair enzymes, and modulates apoptosis (programmed cell death).[48] The science and understanding of how stress affects cancer is still not fully developed, although many researchers are now actively looking at the stress response within the context of cancer control.

This double-edged force of stress is further evidenced when we look at the response of a stress-related gene, ATF3, and breast cancer cells. In general, the ATF3 gene protects the body from harm by causing normal cells to commit suicide if there is a risk they have become permanently damaged by the stressful conditions—for example, if the cells have been affected by cancer or infections. Therefore, ATF3 is a useful defender in early stages. The problem is that cancer cells can switch on ATF3 within immune system cells, making these cells malfunction and resulting in cancers spreading further. Researchers are now looking at ways to harness this stress response to fight cancer cells.

After my experience with Robert and Raewyn, I took time to trawl through all the current literature and scientific studies on stress and cancer. We now know this much is true: there have been no studies that prove stress causes cancer, but there are plenty that show that once you have cancer, stress makes it inherently worse.

Conclusion

Arthur C. Clarke wrote a short story called "The Nine Billion Names of God," in which a Tibetan monk asks a computer firm for help with compiling all the possible names of God—a task they believe was the real purpose of mankind.[49] They wish to write all these names with an alphabet of nine letters, estimate that they will have nine billion permutations, and think the task will last several lifetimes. But with the help of a computer (Mark V Automatic Sequence Computer), a diesel generator (which the monks already use to power their prayer wheels), and some engineers, they reckon the task could be done in a mere one hundred days.[50] As the engineers undertake the task, they realize that the monks actually believe that once the task is done, the world will end, as God will shut down everything. Though they do not truly believe in this, the computer engineers nevertheless sneak away as the computer completes the task and look up to see stars, one by one, turning themselves off.

This story always makes me think of genes. Our genes are like biological stars, predictors of our health heredity, but here's the real parallel—stars used to guide human songlines, our ancestral footprint, and genes are our health blueprint. Like the monks in the story, we may have used computers to map our genetic codes completely, but this self-knowledge only helps mankind if we can live well, not puffed up with illusions of immortality. Genes, like stars in Clarke's story, are nonjudgmental and can turn themselves on and off. Happiness is always there, but sometimes, because of darkness within our genes, we may not see it. Genes may be powerful, but it is our actions that determine their outcome. As John Green wrote in *The Fault in Our Stars*: "It's a metaphor, see: You put the killing thing right between your teeth, but you don't give it the power to do its killing."[51]

Thierry Steimer researched a book published in 1878 (*Physiologie des passions*) by Charles Letourneau, who defined emotions as "passions of a short duration" and concluded that such feelings were "intimately linked with organic life," and either result in an "abnormal excitation of the nervous network," which induces changes in heart rate and secretions, or interrupt "the normal relationship between the peripheral nervous system and the brain."[52] Letourneau also noted "the strong cerebral excitation" that accompanies emotions probably only concerned "certain groups of conscious cells" in the brain and "must necessitate a considerable increase of blood flow in the cell regions involved."[53] What a wonderful summary of the stress response all those years ago.

If anxiety and stress can cause a multitude of illnesses, can the power of positivity overcome the stress response and reduce illnesses? Understanding the scaredy-cat genes is to understand how memories of rewarding and fearful events are stored in the brain's hippocampus.

Conducting an experiment on mice, researchers put male mice in three situations—in a cage with a female (rewarding), alone in a cage (neutral), and alone in a cage immobilized or tethered (stressful).[54] When the mice were happy with a mate, a blue light was shone on the cage. Later, as this process was repeated, mice developed a memory of stressful events or recall of a happy environment. When mice were feeling depressed, the shining of a light source ended up activating neurons that reversed this depression. Therefore, anxiety that is a stress response can lead to depression when the ability of an individual to remember the path to happiness is disrupted.

Therein lies the solution to therapy—positive psychology training that includes understanding memories of happiness (and sadness). This approach, which seeks to improve well-being, rather than the drug therapy model of reducing suffering, is, in my view, more desirable. As Martin Seligman, psychologist and author of *Learned Optimism* and other self-help books, puts this method succinctly:

> It's a matter of ABC: When we encounter Adversity, we react by thinking about it. Our thoughts rapidly congeal into Beliefs. These beliefs may become so habitual we don't even realize we have them unless we stop to focus on them. And they don't just sit there idly; they have Consequences.[55]

When studies were done on positivity and the response of the immune system, they found that optimism can have both positive and negative immune correlates. Optimists indeed fared better as long as their systems responded; if there was a lack of response, the optimists were not immune to disappointment. This is what researchers call the *disappointment hypothesis*. Optimists had higher cortisol levels after tasks, and that made them handle stress better.

Why is the power of positive thought so important? At the University of Pennsylvania, Seligman has even devised a test that can measure a person's level of optimism. Many companies have used his methods as a benchmark when hiring people—for example, in sales jobs, Seligman's optimists outsold the pessimists by more than twice as much. When an optimist fails, Seligman explains, they attribute failure to something they can change, not a weakness they are struggling to overcome. This is what defines those who have found success in the face of adversity.[56]

Ultimately, it is clear that the answer (from scientific research) to the question of whether optimism is good for immunity is a resounding yes![57]

Thus, stress for a short period may indeed give your system a workout; it is chronic stress that becomes harmful. This is why the stress response is inherently neither good nor bad—it is what it is. What evolved as a response to danger has been allowed to morph into something dangerous due to our inadequate coping mechanisms and our overreliance on drugs. As Deepak Chopra noted in *The Book of Secrets: Unlocking the Hidden Dimensions of Your Life*:

> On some dimension or other, every event in life can be causing only one of two things: either it is good for you, or it is bringing up what you need to look at in order to create good for you. Evolution is win-win . . . life is self-correcting.[58]

In June 2016, I was invited to speak at the Dalkey Book Festival in Dublin alongside Ian Robertson, professor of psychology at Trinity College Dublin and founding director of the Trinity College Institute of Neuroscience. Ian views stress as a drug—too little may not be effective, too much (an overdose) is bad, but in the right doses, it may well hit the sweet spot and prove extremely useful. But using stress as a positive force needs some mind training.

The trick is to develop mechanisms to make sure the feeling of stress is acute and does not last for long. The secret is in not worrying about things one cannot control, like what others say about you or unrealistic expectations and other people's actions; similarly, there is no point worrying about things within your control, like jobs or relationships—if they are not working out, you can change them. This is the Tibetan Buddhist approach, and the Dalai Lama summarizes this power of positivity well: "If a problem is fixable, if a situation is such that you can do something about it, then there is no need to worry. If it's not fixable, then there is no help in worrying. There is no benefit in worrying whatsoever."[59]

If anxiety is just an elaborate form of fear, how can we train our minds to free themselves from such symptoms? In 1926, Ivan Pavlov, who had studied conditioned reflexes in dogs by demonstrating that, at the sound of a metronome, a trained dog would salivate, noted that, after a flood in Leningrad, these dogs had developed "learning impairment."[60] The stress response caused by the floods had led to "chronic inhibition." Studies have also shown that babies handled lovingly in the period immediately after birth showed positive effects on their memory later on.[61]

When researchers in India studied rats placed under stressful conditions, they found that the rats started acting anxiously even when they weren't being constrained.[62] Even when they had room to move in a maze, they would prefer dark corners rather than getting out and exploring bright, open spaces. When brain scans were done on these rats, they demonstrated an increase in the size of their amygdalas, almond-shaped structures that are implicated in both fear and pleasure responses. Therefore, it must follow that shrinking the amygdala may be a way to train the brain to reduce stress.

Writing in *The Connection*, a blog and documentary about mind-body medicine, Shannon Harvey interviewed neuroscientist Dr. Sara Lazar of Harvard University, who studied people with no prior knowledge of meditation to see if it would shrink the amygdala. Harvey writes:

Dr. Lazar put people who had never meditated through an eight-week meditation program and observed that the amygdala of her subjects actually got smaller. They also reported less stress and greater feelings of peace.[63]

Meditation works. Irrespective of the genetic hand we've been dealt, we have the ability to express our genes and modify our responses to stress. Mindfulness and meditation, or mindful meditation—creating awareness of present-moment experience with a kinder, nonjudgmental stance—and shifting perception to not allow situations to get to you have also been shown to increase gray matter density in brain scans. The hippocampus, which affects learning and emotions, and the insula, the part of the brain linked to awareness, both showed increases in gray matter on brain scans. Such changes are not confined to humans. Studies have shown that meditative music even improves cognitive behavior in snails.[64] Perhaps it isn't surprising that men and snails have the same stress responses because, after all, isn't evolution just a massive slugfest for survival of a species? Nature takes great care in overseeing this war, and with great precision, it has placed incremental genetic gateposts, calculating each species' ability to cope under duress. But even reluctant warriors can overcome saber-toothed cats by strategy or nous. Chance plays very little part. The stress response is a well-established evolutionary strategy and to overcome the negative effects, we need to be tactical. To win the war against worry, we have to live in the moment and acknowledge that saber-tooth cats have long been extinct—and this is where meditation, not medication, can become both the means and the end.

Reader Rx: Meditation

Focus on managing your stress levels. Keep in mind that acute stress is not necessarily a bad thing if it remains acute. The danger to your health comes when the stress lingers and becomes chronic. There are many methods of meditation, and some methods advocate the use of a mantra, or words you repeat during meditation; here are some simple steps:[65]

- Choose your mantra (any two words).
- Find a quiet and comfortable place to sit or lie down.
- Close your eyes, and practice deep relaxing breathing.
- Repeat your mantra, even if silently.
- If your mind wanders, so be it. Don't try to rein it in; just repeat the mantra.
- After about thirty minutes, you can stop repeating the mantra, and with daily practice, you may not need a mantra to reach meditative bliss.

Key Points

1. Stress response evolved as a mechanism to deal with our fight-or-flight responses.
2. We live in relatively safe times, yet this stress response has become overused by our information overload.
3. Stress can cause a multitude of illnesses and suppress immune systems when it happens over an extended period.
4. Stress is a double-edged sword—short bursts of stress can be beneficial, but long-term stress is dangerous.
5. Anxiety is basically an overactive stress response.
6. There is very little proven science behind antidepressant drugs, even if they are effective for some people.
7. Mind training can help us harness the power of stress by making sure it remains short-term and positive.
8. Optimists perform better, work harder, and have better immunity.

4

THE FAT GENES: SKINNY BRAINS AND FAT GUTS

All men live enveloped in whale-lines. All are born with halters
round their necks; but it is only when caught in the swift,
sudden turn of death, that mortals realize the silent,
subtle, ever-present perils of life.

—Moby Dick

Melville's classic novel *Moby Dick* is also simply referred to as *The Whale*. Whales and other large animals have been a source of fascination, food, and fear due to their sheer size. Sperm whales weigh on average thirty-three thousand pounds; an African elephant weighs around twelve thousand pounds. Whales have a brain size of around fifteen pounds; African elephants have a brain size of around ten pounds. One of the first people to record the weight of an elephant's brain (and other organs) was Allen Mullen of Dublin who wrote a report to the Royal Society in 1690.

On June 17, 1681, an elephant kept in a booth for public viewing succumbed to an accidental fire. As few people in Dublin had seen it when it was alive (due to the price, this kind of activity was the privilege of the rich), a crowd gathered and tried to take away some part of the animal as souvenirs. Allen Mullen rushed to the scene and, aided by a team of butchers, undertook a detailed anatomical dissection of the beast—meticulously recording his findings in a letter to Sir William Petty of the Royal Society, and the chemist and philosopher Robert Boyle. Signed simply "A. M.," it was a remarkable postmortem. Noting the presence of air cells in the sinuses of the elephant's head, he surmised:

> This I am told weigh'd fifty pound, or near upon it. I suppose therefore, that the aforesaid Cells were form'd to obviate that great inconveniency, that is, the Heads being too heavy for the Body . . . The *Cerebellum*, was like that of a Man, only that it was bigger; both it and the *Cerebrum* [w]eig[h]'d Ten Pounds.[1]

Ten pounds! Is that all the brain of an elephant weighs? It must be some kind of record, right? Actually, it isn't. *Acanthonus armatus*, a fish with a tiny brain and large ears, the rather unfortunately named bony-eared assfish, has the smallest brain-to-body ratio.[2] An elephant has a brain-to-body-size ratio of 0.17 percent, a sperm whale has a brain that is only 0.023 percent of its body weight, and a human brain accounts for 2 percent of body weight. Here's the scary thing that happens when humans develop more fat—our brains begin to shrink. Studies have shown a 2.4 percent decrease in brain parenchymal volume (the functional portion of the brain, as opposed to support structure) is observed in obese individuals compared to those with a normal body mass index (BMI).[3] Therefore, studies show that in very obese individuals, over a ten-year period, the executive capabilities of their brains decreased.

Next, these researchers looked at the types of fatness—central or abdominal fat is normally measured by the waist-to-hip ratio and high-risk waist sizes are generally greater than 40 inches in men and greater than 34 inches in women. A higher waist-to-hip reduces the volume of the hippocampus—the part of the brain that controls emotion, memory, and also automatic functions of the brain, such as cardiac and respiratory functions. Further, more corpulent bellies lead to immediate memory loss and a higher risk of dementia thirty years later.[4]

As we've seen so far in this book, evolution and health are an admixture of genes and environment. There is a fatness gene—in other words, a genetic component of obesity has been identified within variants of the fat mass and obesity-associated (FTO) gene. People who carry different high-risk alleles of this FTO gene have a far greater risk of fatness. For example, an extra copy of the A allele results in an average 2.6-pound higher weight gain and a one-centimeter greater waist circumference.[5] Here's the clincher—carriers of the obesity-related gene variants had an 8 percent reduction in brain tissue in the bilateral frontal lobe, and a 12 percent reduction in the bilateral occipital lobe compared to those without the gene.[6] What this means is that we already know increased fatness shrinks the brain, but when the FTO gene is added to the mix, the effect of reduction in brain size is even greater. And while health authorities tell us that human populations are getting fatter, the science behind that means that our brains are getting skinnier!

Strangely, I must say I first thought about this relationship between brains and guts after I opened Baci Lounge, an independent bookstore and café in Auckland, New Zealand (later, expanding alphabetically, we opened a store in Brisbane, Australia). Baci Lounge was featured in *TIME Magazine* in 2008, and even won Auckland's Top Shop award. Baci Lounge was my model of social entrepreneurship and helped fund my school literacy programs in economically disadvantaged areas. To begin with, it was 80 percent bookstore and 20 percent café. I envisaged a diet of great science writing to chew the fat over, perhaps a spicy biography or a cheesy short story. However, as the decade progressed, people began reading less and eating more, and it ended up 80 percent café and 20 percent bookstore—as the local populace evolved into hobbits with fatter guts and skinnier brains.

How could a book lover like me adjust debts when the heart of the business was failing? I could have made the store work—made debts disappear by running it as a café, even made a small profit—by feeding the hungry hordes. But it was a thirst for the written word that I had hoped to encourage. When old patrons ask me why I shut down my beloved, award-winning Baci Lounge, I say, "Skinny brains, fat guts."

Brain versus gut size is actually one of the most debated aspects of our evolutionary history. According to the expansive-tissue (or skinny brains, fat guts) hypothesis, there is a trade-off between our guts and brain sizes—our stomach or gastrointestinal tracts consume a lot of our energy, and because our brains take up a large portion of our body's energy resources, there must be an inverse relationship between the sizes of our brains and guts—a sort of biological battle for energy sources.

Evolution and the Gut

A research team led by Dr. Ana Navarrete set out to test the gut-brain theory by dissecting a hundred different species of animals and measuring brain size, gut size, and body fat.[7] What they discovered was that brain size indeed correlates negatively with the amount of body fat in most mammals. However, brain size was not linked to the mass of the intestines or liver, as these organs are great consumers of energy.

Primates have thrice the brain size of other mammals, and humans have almost thrice the brain size of primates. The human brain accounts for 2 percent of adult body mass, yet consumes 65 percent of its energy in a baby and around 25 percent of its energy in an adult. By age two, babies have a brain 80 percent the size of an adult brain.

Over the past 2.5 million years, as primitive humans began to improve their daily diets and began consuming higher-energy foods, this resulted in a reduction in stomach sizes. A key part of the expansive-tissue hypothesis, therefore, is that the energy needed for brain expansion in early humans was compensated for by a reduction in gut size. Perhaps now, we are heading in an opposite direction—evolutionarily weaker but a digestively delicious path.

We know that primitive humans of the Australopithecus species emerged from the common ancestor we share with the bonobo apes and chimpanzees. Therefore, scientists decided to study bonobo apes to understand the evolution and expression of human fat genes. They found that these bonobo apes had almost no fat. When dissections were carried out on bonobos that had died of natural causes, the average male had a body fat of 0.005 percent of their body mass while in females it made up 3.6 percent. But research suggests that australopithecines had a body fat of around 2 percent in males and 8 percent to 10 percent in females. The theory is that as these humans began walking longer distances, away from traditional food sources, fat emerged as a way to store energy. The reason women have more fat is because their fat varies with their reproductive cycles, which increases their chances of producing babies.

Fast-forward to Homo erectus and Homo sapiens, and females gradually gained more fat—in our species, females need 12 to 14 percent body fat to maintain fertility. As we discussed earlier, as humans walked greater distances, they developed larger brains. To nourish babies of this new species with larger brains, women needed to have more fat stores. While the appropriate body fat levels have remained the same, modern humans, in contrast, have a 15 percent global obesity rate and two-thirds of the American population is overweight.

The average human female has a body fat of 25 to 30 percent, while the average male has around 18 to 24 percent.

We can now see why we developed fat stores, as they were efficient energy stores in times of hunger or famine. For example, a lean, 165-pound man typically has over one hundred thousand calories stored in the form of fat. If we had to store this energy purely as carbohydrate (glycogen, the storage form of carbs, is less energy dense), the man would end up weighing upward of 275 pounds.

Leptin, the hormone we discussed earlier, tells our brains that we have fat available in storage units. But the problem is the more fat that is stored, the higher the leptin levels in the blood. This resets the brain into thinking that this higher leptin level is normal. The brain is only wired to detect sudden drops that could indicate a famine. This makes evolutionary sense because, for millions of years, we have been storing fat so we can use it when there is a very good reason.

A human's fat cell count remains the same from birth through life. However, it must be noted that this fatty adipose tissue is capable of fifteen fold expansion. Also, there are two types of fat in mammals—white fat and brown fat. The former is designed to store energy (what humans developed during periods of food scarcity), and the latter dissipates energy and generates heat—this is what hibernating animals use in winter.

Recently scientists in Gothenburg, Sweden, discovered two different types of brown fat cells—one which young people have as "baby fat," which disappears during adolescence.[8] Many teams are now searching for ways to switch white into brown fat, as the latter would lower the risk of diabetes and heart disease. In 2012, Bruce Spiegelman, professor of cell biology at Harvard Medical School and the Dana-Farber Cancer Institute, reported that irisin, a muscle hormone, could switch white into brown fat.[9] People were skeptical if such a compound existed and called this a study a fraud. Spiegelman's team defended their findings convincingly; however, other studies have also shown that genes like PRDM16 play a major part in this fat conversion, and these have future implications regarding our ability to reduce the risk of complications from having too much fat.

Researchers have now found that when it comes to brain weight, it is more the neuron count that matters. The human brain weighs about three pounds, but the cerebral cortex of the brain contains approximately sixteen billion neurons; in contrast, an elephant brain weighs ten pounds but contains only around five billion neurons. Humans and apes like chimps have almost the same gene sequence, but humans have DNA sequences called *human accelerated regions* (HARs) that cause more neuronal growth; therefore, when modern humans emerged in Africa two hundred thousand years ago, their brains had tripled in size due to the growth of more nerve cells.

Thus, both larger brains and fat storage may actually be measures to help ward off starvation. Brain sizes increased as humans became two legged and, therefore, more mobile, while fat stores were useful during periods when food sources were scarce. This explains why, for example, this evolutionary strategy did not work for birds because flying expends a lot more energy than walking and therefore creatures of flight ended up with a, well, bird brain. Because of the need to battle gravity, even skinny birds can't develop bigger brains.

Paleolithic Diet: Then and Now

The Paleolithic period refers to the Old Stone Age, the beginning of the period about 2.5 million years ago when primitive humans began to use tools and which extended to the upper Paleolithic period, which began as recently as forty thosuand years ago—although recently a team of researchers found 3.3-million-year-old stone tools from Lomekwi 3, West Turkana, Kenya, suggesting that primitive humans used hand tools much earlier than previously thought.

As a physician, I am often asked about the Paleo diet. The premise behind the Paleo diet is eating as primitive humans did. This is because, on one hand, it is true that our overall genetic makeup differs very little from that of our ancestors fifty thousand to one hundred thousand years ago. On the other hand, as I mentioned earlier, evolution has been rapid in the last fifty thousand years—gene expressions have changed due to different environments and exposure to microbes. How did this happen? Because, as discussed in the previous chapter, our lifestyles lead to gene expression. Gene expression means the genetic information in our genes is used to produce new products—proteins or even bits of RNA, which are companions of DNA in coding, decoding, regulation, and expression of genes. Therefore, while our genetic codes may have changed little, the effects of our diets and migration led to many new products of gene expression, a speeding up of evolution. Our gene expressions have ballooned, just like our appetites, and we've moved away from having to coexist with others. Our genes ended up cleverly engineered for our species, and were scattered around without bias. However, irrespective of what our genetics forecasts, there is always hope in genetic karma—our ability to influence our gene codes by our actions.

The truth is, although we may romanticize the past and sometimes behave like cavemen, we are no longer Paleo humans, even if their less-processed diets have certain benefits. For a start, we don't have access to many of the plants and meats they ate, so let's stop kidding ourselves about the great marketing myth that is the Paleo diet. If we ate a truly Paleo diet, we'd miss out on much of the good tinkering our bodies have done in expressing good genes due to new beneficial food sources from modern diets. Marlene Zuk, evolutionary biologist, calls this the "Paleofantasy" in her book under the same name:

"Paleofantasies" call to mind a time when everything about us—body, mind, and behavior—was in sync with the envi-

ronment . . . but no such time existed . . . We and every other living thing have always lurched along in evolutionary time, with the inevitable trade-offs that are a hallmark of life.[10]

For a start, how do we know what primitive humans ate? Essentially, we are what we eat, or we end up that way. Stable carbon, nitrogen, and sulfur isotopes are analyzed in fossilized soft and mineralized tissues, such as bone, and these help us reconstruct diets. Whole bone pieces are soaked in acetone to remove potential contaminants before they are demineralized. Collagen is then extracted by soaking samples in hydrochloric acid until it is demineralized. It is then gelatinized and undergoes an ultrafiltration process. Then, the samples are ready for isotope analyses. Such stable isotope ratios do not reproduce exact menus or differentiate between good or bad eating habits; however, they are remarkably able to distinguish between broad food categories: meat versus plants, land versus marine protein sources, and so on. Think *CSI* for an anthropology nerd.

Primitive hunter-gatherers, at least in the early part of the Stone Age, were reliant on meat for the majority of their diet—at least 50 percent of their calorie intake was composed of meat. It is estimated that in the last one hundred thousand years, cholesterol intake was around 500 milligrams per day. Yet the average cholesterol for hunter-gatherers was 101–141 mg/dL, far less than the modern human. The average lion supposedly sleeps for around twenty hours a day, and even with all this lack of exercise or burning of calories, and an exclusively meat-eating diet, it still has blood cholesterol levels around 30 mg/dL less than humans! So there must be factors other than pure cholesterol intake involved. And unlike humans, lions are exclusive carnivores and sensitive to lack of certain amino acids like arginine and taurine, which are only found in fresh kill.

There is some interesting science behind high meat intake and cholesterol levels. Ancient men consumed all edible portions of game

animals, not just muscle, and derived about 35 percent of their total calorie intake from meat (which is higher than what we consider safe these days).

If we look at the Stone Age dietary pattern, we can calculate a cholesterol level with a maximum of 150 mg/dL and a mean of 125 mg/dL. About fifty years ago, the average cholesterol level in the US was 222 mg/dL. After the turn of the millennium, due to the use of statin drugs, the average cholesterol level in the US dropped to 199 mg/dL. Comparative serum cholesterol levels of man and other animals make for interesting reading, as we can compare herbivores, carnivores, and omnivores and see how out-of-kilter modern humans have become:

Species	Serum Cholesterol (mmol/l)	Serum Cholesterol (mg/dL)
Goats	1.4–1.6	52–62
Deer	1.8–2.5	68–96
Pigs	1.9–2.5	73–98
Lions	3.8-4.4	147–170
Snow leopards	3.2–3.4	124–131
Hunter-gatherer humans	2.6–3.7	101–141
Swiss humans (1999–2001)	5.8	222
US humans (2005–2006)	5.2	199

[11]

History and diet patterns of ancient humans show that fat intake has very little to do with actual serum cholesterol levels. When it comes to fat, it is the type that matters.

From a chemical point of view, a fat is saturated if it contains maximal levels of hydrogen atoms and is unsaturated if some hydrogen atoms are missing and replaced by double bonds between the carbon atoms. Further, if unsaturated fats contain one double bond only, they are termed *monounsaturated* (e.g., peanut and olive oils are mostly monounsaturated), and if they contain more than one double bond, they are called polyunsaturated fats (e.g., soybean, sunflower, and salmon oils are mostly polyunsaturated). Most cooking oils are a mix of all these types, with rice bran oil, for example, containing almost equal portions of all these different types of fats. However, when it comes to saturated fats we know this much is true:

- When levels of saturated fat are maintained in the diet and do not change daily, it does not seem to affect serum cholesterol concentrations.
- When we compare the roe deer that our Paleolithic ancestors ate with our modern choice of beef cows, the deer has 7 percent carcass fat as opposed to 40 percent of our beef cattle. And even if we just take muscle meat, deer and antelope have 14 percent less than commercial beef. Therefore, while Stone Age folk ate more meat, their diet comprised much less saturated fat when compared to modern humans (8 percent versus 12 percent of diets).
- Unsaturated fats that chemically contain at least one double bond in the trans configuration are what we refer to as trans fats. These are high in margarine and hydrogenated oils used in processed foods like cakes and fast food like burgers and fries. Small amounts of trans fats do occur in nature in beef and butter. However, in the Paleolithic period, trans fat intake was less than half of what the average human consumes today. This is what makes processed meats unhealthy.

Changes in levels of polyunsaturated fat levels are also worth looking at as human evolution unfolded—especially the ratio between omega-3 and omega-6 fatty acids that are important components of cell membranes and, therefore, are involved in regulating blood pressure and inflammatory processes. The human body, both for prehistoric humans and today's population, is capable of producing all the fatty acids it needs except for two: linoleic acid (LA), an omega-6 fatty acid, and alpha-linolenic acid (ALA), an omega-3 fatty acid. ALA and LA are found in plant and seed oils. Although the levels of LA are usually much higher than those of ALA, rapeseed oil and walnut oil are still very good sources of the latter. Both of these fatty acids are needed for growth and repair but can also be used to make other fatty acids (e.g., arachidonic acid (AA) that is present in egg yolks can be formed from LA). Likewise about 8 to 20 percent of ALA is converted to eicosapentaenoic acid (EPA), which has been shown to have cardio-protective abilities and is found in fish oils. Flaxseed oil, for example, is rich in omega-3 oil but not as efficient as fish oil in converting this to EPA or docosahexaenoic acid (DHA). The latter is found as a structural component in the skin, brain, and testicles that ancient humans did not discard from their diets.

Even in our more recent past, humans' consumption of meat leaned more toward marine, rather than land, animals—the opposite of today's diets. In August 1999, the remains of a preserved ice body were recovered from a retreating glacier in the Tatshenshini-Alsek Park, British Columbia. Radiocarbon dating calibrated that the remains, named Kwädąy Dän Ts'ìnchi (which translates to "long ago person found"), were of a person who had lived between 1670 and 1850 AD, predating European contact in this region. Molecular fingerprinting and compound-specific carbon isotope analysis were performed on individual lipids extracted from his bone and skin. Analyses suggested this person consumed meat. However, most unusual was the presence of long-chain hydroxy FAs (LCHFAs), 10- and 12-hydroxyeicosanoic acid and 10- and 12-hydroxydocosanoic acid, in the bone—the latter indicated a largely marine-based diet, even though this remote location was more than fifty miles inland.[12]

There is plenty of evidence that over the last 150 years, intake of omega-6 have increased and intake of omega-3 have decreased with the increase in heart disease. Therefore, it is worth looking at the omega-3 and omega-6 ratios of Paleo humans. Purslane (*Portulaca oleracea*), often called pigweed or verdolaga, is an ancient succulent that was widely consumed by primitive humans. Interestingly, it has eight times the ALA when compared to common vegetables consumed these days (carrots, beans, peas, spinach, tomato, etc.). Analyses of ancient diets reveal that human beings evolved on a diet with a ratio of omega-6 to omega-3 essential fatty acids (EFA) of approximately one to one, whereas, in Western diets, the ratio is approximately fifteen to one.

Reports have suggested that a lower omega-6 to omega-3 ratio in women reduces the risk of breast cancer and Alzheimer's disease.[13] It is well known that processed meats such as bacon contain high LDL cholesterol; however, a recent WHO report found that eating fifty grams of processed meat per day (two strips of bacon) also increased the risk of bowel cancer by 18 percent.[14] Further, an omega-6 to omega-3 ratio of between two and three to one suppressed inflammation in patients with rheumatoid arthritis, and a ratio of five to one had a beneficial effect on patients with asthma, whereas a ratio of ten to one had many adverse health consequences. And all the medical conditions listed above are becoming increasingly common in modern industrialized diets. Therefore, a return to unprocessed traditional diets may be in order.

In his book *Survival of the Fattest: The Key to Human Brain Evolution*, Stephen Cunnane describes how humans moving to a shore-based diet was a recipe for fatness. Suddenly our diet contained shellfish, fish, marsh plants, and frogs—things that didn't involve running after or spearing. Fishing from the shore was a relatively sedentary pastime that needed less leg movement than previously and, therefore, increased our fatness as a species.[15]

The interesting thing with omega-3 is that it protects against a lot of obesity-related diseases like diabetes and heart disease, even if it does not prevent fatness. Meaning it *is* possible to be fat and healthy. Scientists from the Fred Hutchinson Cancer Research Center in Seattle studied Yup'ik Eskimos in Alaska—these people ate twenty times the omega-3 of the average American diet, since their meat was largely marine, especially salmon. When these researchers measured their BMI, they found something interesting—they had the same number of obese individuals as the general population; however, their prevalence of diabetes was less than half of the US population (3.3 percent versus 7.7 percent).[16]

The chart on the next page illustrates the different levels of saturated and unsaturated fats contained in commonly used cooking oils.

To summarize, the less saturated fat one eats, the better (especially in our modern varied diets); however, when it comes to polyunsaturated fats, omega-3 is more important than omega-6, as ancient human diets reveal. Unsaturated fats can be found naturally (in dairy and meat), but artificial trans fats that are used to thicken oils such as margarine or those found in processed foods are worse. Therefore, when we think we are following a Paleo diet, we aren't, as many of those plant sources are no longer available and the meat we farm is not as lean.

When it comes to saturated fats, the types vary—some may be long chain (more than twelve carbon atoms) or medium chain (under twelve carbon atoms). Chocolate contains stearic acid, a long-chain fatty acid (LCFA)—chocolate or cocoa butter raises LDL cholesterol only about one-quarter as much as butter, even though both are about 60 percent saturated fat; this is because stearic acid is shown to have a neutral effect on cholesterol.

A study published by Dr. James Pottala in *Neurology* looked at one thousand women and their omega-3 indices, measuring the con-

Dietary Guidelines for Americans[17]

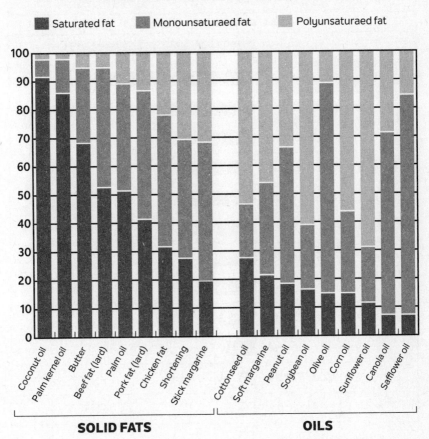

- ■ Saturated fat
- ■ Monounsaturaed fat
- ■ Polyunsaturaed fat

SOLID FATS **OILS**

centration of their omega-3 fatty acids as a percentage of all fatty acids on their red blood cells. The results were astounding—omega-3 acids *increased* brain size. The hippocampus, the area of the brain related to cognitive function, was also significantly smaller in women with lower omega-3 indices, linking to a higher risk of Alzheimer's dementia. We have come full circle: *fat brains, skinny guts.*

The chart on the next page shows the comparative omega-3 levels contained in fish meat:[18]

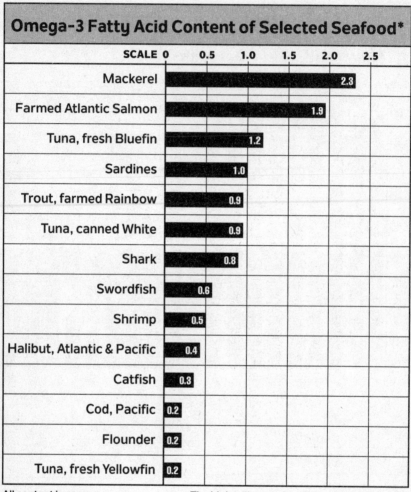

Omega-3 Fatty Acid Content of Selected Seafood*

SCALE	0	0.5	1.0	1.5	2.0	2.5
Mackerel					2.3	
Farmed Atlantic Salmon					1.9	
Tuna, fresh Bluefin			1.2			
Sardines			1.0			
Trout, farmed Rainbow		0.9				
Tuna, canned White		0.9				
Shark		0.8				
Swordfish		0.6				
Shrimp		0.5				
Halibut, Atlantic & Pacific		0.4				
Catfish		0.3				
Cod, Pacific	0.2					
Flounder	0.2					
Tuna, fresh Yellowfin	0.2					

All content in grams · The higher the number, the better the content
Scale is per 100 grams, raw
Source: USDA Nutrient Database for Standard/Reference, Release 16 (2003)
*EPA and DHA

And, when we examine carbohydrates, 85 percent of modern carbohydrate intakes are from cereals. "Added sugars" alone account for 15 percent. Humans in Africa in the past (fifty thousand years ago) obtained 35 percent of their energy from carbohydrates, but almost all of this came from fruits and vegetables, not from cereals, as the latter were too labor-intensive to make. Honey was the only "added sugar" in Stone Age times and accounted for only 2 to 3 percent of energy.

We often speak of the importance of dietary fiber, but we don't differentiate between insoluble and soluble fiber—the former aids bowel movement; the latter reduces cholesterol levels. In the Paleolithic diet, soluble fiber was from fruits and vegetables, whereas, today, we derive most of our fiber from cereals. Ancestral fiber intake is estimated at five times that of the average diet in affluent countries.[19] Less than 5 percent of Americans maintain recommended dietary levels of fiber. And any fiber consumed is largely cereal based from foods such as rice, wheat, and corn. In ancient diets, pulses were much more common—indeed, pulse crops or legumes such as broad beans, chickpeas, and lentils are one of the most concentrated sources of dietary fiber.

Reconstructing our genetic pasts can be tricky for humans. We behave as though we are precious objects that must be saved at the expense of other creatures. Destroying the planetary house we were born into does not seem to cause us sufficient alarm. We live lives full of busy intensity, divided by land and country, creating processed foods and minds, without enough time spent on contemplating the history of our species. For example, Western diets are deficient in omega-3 fatty acids and have excessive amounts of omega-6 fatty acids compared with the diet human beings evolved on—and more importantly, this is how our genetic patterns were established.

The problem with our genetic past is that there is no escaping it. Our genes accompany us everywhere. Doing what is right by our genetic pasts allows us the unadulterated freedom of good health. If we were to follow prehistoric dietary patterns, a diet that we were suited to from an evolutionary point of view, we would eliminate trans fat in our diets, eat more fiber, make sure our omega-3 to omega-6 ratios are almost one, and reduce refined or added sugar to under 5 percent of our energy needs. But we'd still be modern humans adapting our diets to as close to what nature intended, not prehistoric Paleo people.

Guts and Brains in the Modern Age

When I was around eleven, in the late seventies, my father asked me to cut down my egg consumption after reading an article in a medical journal. What would happen if I ate a dozen eggs a day? I asked, having read that some weightlifters consumed such quantities.

"You could die of heart disease," my father explained in simple but scary language, easily understood by a child. A few year earlier, the US dietary guidelines for fat had been released and had recommended the following: trim fat to one-third of total daily calories and cut saturated fat—from red meat and dairy products like milk, eggs, and cheese in particular—down to one-tenth of total calories. When I look at those recommendations today, I am astounded at the lack of science. There was no actual linkage to deaths it would prevent or any explanation how those numbers were arrived at.

As a physician and scientist, I understand the imperfection of statistics. Because the United States had such a high rate of heart disease, everyone jumped on the fat bandwagon. Advice about fat was speedily adopted by doctors everywhere, and repeated as gospel truth. But populations were being asked to make massive dietary changes to their fat consumption with no real factual basis. In an era when universities were beginning to look at the mathematics of things like poetry and dance, this was scientific satire at its best—at its worst, a terrible industry myth.

Zoe Harcombe, a researcher at University of the West of Scotland, reviewed these guidelines in the journal *OpenHeart* and noted: "The bottom line is that there wasn't evidence for those guidelines to be introduced . . . One of the most important things that should have underpinned the guidelines is sound nutritional knowledge, and that was distinctly lacking."[20] The article concluded:

"Dietary recommendations were introduced for 220 million US and 56 million UK citizens by 1983, in the absence of supporting evidence from randomized-controlled trials."[21]

It seems as though the same situation applies to low-fat (low-energy) diets. When it comes to fatness and dieting, specific diets don't seem to matter. In a large meta-analysis—a review of several studies—the authors wrote:

A meta-analysis of randomized, controlled trials that compared rapid weight loss (achieved with very-low-energy diets) with slower weight loss (achieved with low-energy diets—i.e., 800 to 1200 kcal per day) at the end of short-term follow-up (<1 yr) and long-term follow-up (≥1 year) showed that, despite the association of very-low-energy diets with significantly greater weight loss at the end of short-term follow-up (16.1 percent of body weight lost, vs. 9.7 percent with low-energy diets), there was no significant difference between the very-low-energy diets and low-energy diets with respect to weight loss at the end of long-term follow-up.[22]

I guess the message here is one of common sense. Diets don't work. Period. Low fat, high fat, low energy, high energy—it is better to consider everything we ingest as a food source, as we have to eat on a day-to-day basis forever. Most diets have peaks and valleys in the media. We know certain things are really bad for us, like trans fats and refined sugar. Otherwise, food groups like carbohydrates, proteins, and fats meet in our stomachs in gastric collisions. In accordance with well-known laws of metabolism, they are broken down and carried off to different cells, creating energy that allows our bodies and minds to function.

George Eliot wrote in *Middlemarch*: "It's an uncommonly dangerous thing to be left without any padding against the shafts of disease."[23] So can one be fat and healthy, notwithstanding the brain shrinkage that occurs, if he is fat for a long period of time?

A few years ago, I turned on the TV to hear Governor Chris Christie of New Jersey describe himself as "basically the healthiest fat guy you've ever seen."[24] This begs a scientific question: are some humans destined to be bigger, or is it within their control? It turns out that our fat cell count is set at childhood and remains constant—if we gain weight, our adipocytes (fat cells) become larger. After bariatric weight-loss surgery, the fat cells shrink in size, but their overall population is maintained. Kirsty Spalding and others from the Karolinska Institute of Sweden found that in obese adults, this expansion of fat cells begins earlier or ends later than in normal subjects.[25] In general, fat babies become fat adults.[26]

Human infant fatness is quite staggering when we consider average birth weights—a baby elephant seal weighs about 85 pounds, yet has only 2 percent fat at birth; a cat weighs 0.26 pounds, and contains 1.8 percent fat; whereas human babies weigh an average 6.6 pounds, yet have 15 percent body fat.[27] While fat was originally thought to be merely insulation, we now know that baby fat is far more complex and that this energy store helps ward off adversity and infections. I should know.

I was born so prematurely that I was whisked off to one of the few centers in England equipped to deal with tiny preterm infants. In those days, my parents were told (as were many other parents in similar situations) not to let others know that I had been born—that way, if I succumbed to sickness due to my immature lungs, the sadness and disappointment would be only theirs.

Perhaps such adversity creates a fighting spirit. As I went into my warm incubator, laid down gently by nurses, my future could not be denied. By the time I was brought home, I had become so fat that everyone wanted to know what on earth my parents were feeding me. As a medical doctor and evolutionary biologist, I now know that this greater adiposity was for energy storage—an important strategy and a means to improve my chances of survival during the nutritionally and immunologically turbulent period of my early infancy. But as I grew older, I lost most of that fat, especially when I was at boarding school, and I now weigh more or less what I did when I was at university. The only time I gained weight was during a brief period when I drank Coke (Coca-Cola), and we'll be seeing why sugar matters in the next section.

So, while we know fat stores are accumulated in anticipation of famine, are some people genetically predetermined to be fat?

Hormones and Appetite

Studying the genetics of fat would be a good place to start understanding human fatness, surmised Jeffrey Friedman, a molecular geneticist at the Rockefeller University Hospital.[28] He took a look at a study from the summer of 1949, when some very corpulent mice were found and attracted the attention of researchers, as obesity in mice is very rare, except in yellow mice. This led to the finding of a recessive mutation in a gene called *ob* (for obese) that was discovered in mice in 1950 at the Roscoe B. Jackson Laboratory in Maine.

Stunned that a single gene could make mice meaty, Friedman cloned this ob gene and a related gene in humans and ended up discovering a hormone called leptin. Leptin is secreted by adipocytes, essentially fat cells. People with a mutation in this gene lack leptin and tend to overeat, as their brains perceive them to be starving. Giving these people leptin makes them lose weight dramatically. Leptin and a related hormone, amylin, are hot topics in obesity research even today; the latter works for those who are resistant to leptin.

When Shirly Pinto, a postdoctoral scientist at Friedman's lab, studied leptin and the effect on neuronal circuits of the brain, she found that leptin inhibits neurons that encourage the animal to eat and reserve energy and, at the same time, activates neurons that curtail feeding.[29] And it does this by altering the synapses—the points where the cells connect and communicate. In other words, the brains of fat and slim people are wired differently in some cases. However, leptin is still a good measure of fat metabolism.

When leptin isn't there, the person eats; when leptin arrives, it fights the person for his food and allows him to settle for half the usual amount. There is a lot of talking between them and exchanges of neuronal and cellular signals. The two may be wary of each other, and little biochemical arguments do occur, but ultimately a natural balance is struck, and it is this unlikely intimacy that defines the machinations of our human bodies. However, leptin has a doppelgänger, ghrelin, that increases appetite—to simplify, leptin is a hormone made by fat cells that decreases appetite, whereas ghrelin is a hormone that increases appetite, and both play a part in maintenance of our body weight.

The effect of sugar on leptin levels has recently gained wide prominence. Sugar induces leptin resistance and, therefore, ends up having the same effect in causing obesity. University of California, San Francisco, pediatric endocrinologist Robert Lustig feels that the increase in obesity over the last thirty years is the result of one thing: increased amounts of sugar in our diet.[30] Author of the *New York Times* bestseller *Fat Chance: Beating the Odds Against Sugar, Processed Food, Obesity, and Disease,* Lustig suggests that sugar may indeed be the new fat.

But what has sugar got to do with brain size? Recent studies have shown that leptin actually increases brain size. An eighteen-month study at the NIH looked at three people, chosen especially due to a very rare recessive mutation in the ob gene, which is similar to the mutation in obese mice.[31] When these women were given leptin, they lost about 50 percent of their baseline weight, with a preferential loss of fat. But when their bodies were studied with MRI scans, they surprisingly also showed an increase in gray matter concentrations of the brain. And, when four-week-old obese mice were given leptin for two weeks, they also showed a 10 percent increase in brain size.

This increase in weight is partially due to increased cell numbers as indicated by a 19 percent increase in total brain DNA, or in other words—skinny guts, fat brains.

It must be noted that a deficiency of the leptin hormone due to a gene abnormality as a birth defect accounts for fewer than one in two thousand individuals. For most of us, therefore, it is a lack of self-control, and not a gene, that is the culprit. Leptin is essentially a fullness hormone produced by fat cells; therefore, the more fat cells you have, strangely, the more leptin you have (unless you inherit this gene deficiency). This is why crash diets don't work. I am often asked if plastic surgery makes a difference to fat metabolism. Truth be told, liposuction is pretty useless from a metabolic point of view. When you restrict someone's calorie intake severely or suck fat out of them, their leptin levels drop. In response, they get hungrier, thyroid hormones decrease, and their metabolism slows down. This makes them even hungrier and activates hormones that eventually make them pile the weight back on.

Fat and Cholesterol

When it comes to body fat, there seem to be two maladies with far-reaching consequences—corpulence and cholesterol. Studies show that 75 percent of obese children grow up to be obese adults, while only 10 percent of children with healthy weight grow up and maintain a healthy weight.[32]

Earlier we discussed that body fat increases the risk of dementia and reduces brain size. We've been discussing different types of fat and how fat stores emerged as evolution progressed. But how did this fat travel through our system? It was in trying to answer this question that scientists began to understand cholesterol metabolism.

It is clear that for any biochemical change caused by our diets, there are consequences. It was Robert Boyle (the same Boyle who received the letter from "A.M.") who first discovered that animals indeed had a fat transport system. In 1665, Boyle noticed that the lacteals, the intestinal lymphatic vessels, of animals turned milky after a fatty meal and that this emulsion entered the bloodstream via the thoracic duct—a conduit that collects lymph from the body and drains it into some large veins. It would be another century before François Poulletier de la Salle discovered cholesterol in 1769, in bile and gallstones. In 1815, Michel Eugène Chevreul "rediscovered" this fatty substance and named it "cholesterine." In 1924, Simon Henry Gage and Pierre Augustine Fish revisited Boyle's original observations and noted that blood taken from humans after a fatty meal contained tiny particles about one micrometer in diameter (one thousandth of a millimeter or one twenty-five-thousandth of an inch). These particles were named *chylomicrons*.

Essentially, fat is transported by substances called lipoproteins. Lipoproteins also carry cholesterol and protein. Lipoproteins can be divided into LDL, VLDL, and HDL depending on their density, which is also determined by the amount of protein they carry—for example, low-density lipoprotein (LDL) is typically 25 percent protein, whereas high-density lipoprotein (HDL) typically contains 50 percent protein and less fat, and is, therefore, more desirable. The liver, which produces cholesterol regardless of whether our diet contains cholesterol or not, releases another type of lipoprotein, very-low density lipoprotein (VLDL), that contains mostly fatty substances like triglycerides and only 5 to 10 percent protein. When VLDL enters the bloodstream, enzymes break down these triglycerides and this ends up becoming LDL.

Cholesterol is simultaneously the most overused and the most feared word in the medical lexicon. Yet, when it comes to cholesterol, there is more than meets the eye—HDL, LDL, omega-3, polyunsaturated and saturated fats—and there are both good kinds of cholesterol and bad. Get it wrong and you may end up with a heart operation or a plump posterior. So, what is good and bad cholesterol? Let's try and simplify the jargon by referring to information from the American Heart Association:[33]

- LDL cholesterol (the bad cholesterol)—the stuff that clogs arteries, forms plaque, and makes arteries inflexible. This hardening of arteries is known as atherosclerosis. If a clot forms and blocks a narrowed artery, heart attack or stroke can result. Trans fats increase LDL levels.
- HDL cholesterol (the good cholesterol)—HDL cholesterol is considered "good" cholesterol because it helps remove LDL cholesterol from the arteries. Experts believe HDL acts as a scavenger, carrying LDL cholesterol away from the arteries and back to the liver, where it is broken down and passed from the body.
- Triglycerides—Triglycerides are another type of fat, and they're used to store excess energy from your diet. High levels of triglycerides in the blood are also associated with atherosclerosis. Being overweight or obese, physical inactivity, cigarette smoking, excess alcohol consumption, and a diet very high in sugars (more than 60 percent of total calories) also lead to high triglyceride levels.
- Lp(a) or lipoprotein A—Lp(a) consists of an LDL-like particle encoded by a gene that triggers plaque formation and clots. A high level of Lp(a) is a significant risk factor for the premature development of fatty deposits in arteries.

Our total cholesterol scores are calculated using the following equation: HDL + LDL + 20 percent of your triglyceride level.

Remember the obese mice with the abnormal genes? Well, those mice with the abnormal ob genes were sterile but grew to four times the size of their peers.[34] Surprisingly, this rotundity did not seem to affect their life spans. These mice can often be fat but have healthy hearts—the Chris Christies of the murine world—and this is because wild mice are naturally deficient in a plasma gene called CETP, and this makes them carry most of their cholesterol in the good cholesterol variant (HDL) and makes them less prone to their arteries getting clogged.

The Changing Face of Cholesterol Research

Ernest Becker, in *The Denial of Death*, wrote that man "is a creator with a mind that soars out to speculate about atoms and infinity [and] yet, at the same time . . . man is a worm and food for worms."[35] There is no place to investigate atoms (or worms, it seems) like Oxford University, the oldest English-speaking university.

Whenever I'm in the United Kingdom, I make time to visit Keble College, Oxford University, and its able warden, my good friend Jonathan (Sir Jonathan Phillips), who always makes me feel at home. The last time I was there, Jonathan arranged a dinner at the warden's lodgings in my honor but neglected to mention that I was expected to make a speech. It may not have been my best speech, but in true Tractarian Keble tradition, it was a memorable and venerable experience.

At the dinner, I met a young Bengali lad studying worms for insight into human longevity. He had an inquiring mind, and we had a discussion about the work he was involved with. He was studying *Caenorhabditis elegans*, the nonparasitic nematode worm, which has become the new darling of scientists studying organ development, cell death, behavior, and many other biological processes. This one-millimeter soil worm is anatomically simple, easily cultivated in petri dishes, and has a body containing just over one thousand cells, including a 302-cell nervous system. Due to its small size, the entire neuronal circuitry can be studied and possibly reproduced.

It has recently been used to produce models for both neuroscience and robotics. The transparency of the worm's body, the constancy of cell numbers, and the constancy of cell position from individual to individual are unique characteristics that make this worm so heavily studied in medicine and biology.

In 2001, when the details of the human genome were published, everyone was astounded to see that human beings comprised only around thirty thousand genes—far fewer than the originally predicted 150,000. And guess what? *Caenorhabditis elegans*, this tiny worm, contained around nineteen thousand genes. Humans and this worm share around nineteen thousand genes!

Worms ended up becoming entwined in cholesterol research almost by accident because while they need cholesterol to survive, they cannot produce cholesterol themselves. Nematode worms need cholesterol to leave a stage of their life cycle called the *dauer stage*, which is essentially a form of hibernation, so in controlling the worm's access to cholesterol and the various biochemical mediators, scientists are able to study the role of cholesterol. For example, in parasitic worms, molecules derived from cholesterol are actually what tell a worm that it has passed biological borders and is now resident inside a host's body; these worms (and many other parasitic microbes) have cholesterol-sensing receptors. If only humans had these sensors— we'd save a fortune on cardiologists' bills.

Today, it is widely accepted in the medical community that cholesterol worsens heart disease, as do other factors like smoking, high blood pressure, and a lack of exercise. But cholesterol was virtually unknown barely a century ago. In 1913, Nikolaj N. Anitschkow and a colleague, Semen S. Chalatov, conducted a series of experiments on rabbits. Anitschkow and Chalatov began feeding rabbits a diet full of meat, eggs, and milk and noted that the rabbits developed arterial disease, which they believed was similar to human atherosclerosis. To find the offending agent, they began to study each individual component of this diet. Feeding rabbits eggs seemed to cause disease; feeding egg yolks alone did also. Next, they purified cholesterol from egg yolks and dissolved it in sunflower oil. Using this concoction they were again able to produce arterial deposits in these poor rabbits. They then tried sunflower oil alone and found it did not induce disease. Cholesterol was the culprit, they surmised. Feeding cholesterol to the rabbits over time caused deposition of fibrous tissue—fatty streaks became thick and fibrous, further damaging the arterial walls—and this was proportional to the blood cholesterol measurements. Anitschkow surmised:

> The blood of such animals exhibits an enormous increase in cholesterin [cholesterol] content, which in some cases amounts to several times the normal quantity. It may therefore be regarded as certain that in these experimental animals, large quantities of the ingested cholesterin [cholesterol] are absorbed, and that the accumulations of this substance in the tissues can only be interpreted as deposits of lipoids circulating in large quantities in the humors of the body.[36]

Anitschkow hypothesized that cholesterol-laden cells were probably defensive white cells that had engulfed fat; therefore, inflammation must play a part in the generation of arterial plaques. In Anitschkow's original study, no injury had been created to the blood vessels or animal prior to the cholesterol feeding, so his dictum "no atherosclerosis without cholesterol"[37] proved controversial, as many misinterpreted this to mean that Anitschkow wasn't considering other factors that could cause blood vessel injury or inflammation and what he may have noted were just fat deposits and not plaques within the arteries. One of the reasons that the Russians' theories were not initially accepted was that, when Bailey and others from Stanford tried to replicate his experiment using dogs and rats, they failed (because dogs and rats can convert cholesterol into bile acids efficiently, as humans can, unlike rabbits). A rabbit also does not normally have cholesterol in its diet, unlike humans and dogs. These are most likely the reasons why other scientists weren't convinced that this theory of rabbit arteries being lined by cholesterol plaques was relevant.

In 1916, C. D. de Langen, a public health officer in the Dutch East Indies (now Indonesia), noted that natives had much lower cholesterol when compared to the Dutch colonists. The Dutch had a diet rich in meats and butter, while the natives mostly ate rice and vegetables. Anitschkow's experiment on rabbits was not widely known at that time, and de Langen ran his own experiment, using Indonesian local people. He put five Indonesian natives on a "Dutch diet" and found that, at three months, their cholesterol had risen by an average of 27 percent.[38] But given that the research was published in an obscure Dutch journal, the study largely went unnoticed.

After World War II, another Dutchman, J. Groen, commented on the reduction in heart attack rates during the war due to the shortage of food. He conducted experiments comparing a strict vegetarian diet (without dairy) with a diet of meat, butter, and eggs, and found that vegetarians had 25 percent lower blood cholesterol levels.[39] He was meticulous with individual records and noted that certain individuals would not respond in a typical fashion—one person in his study had not raised their blood cholesterol level even on consuming five hundred grams of meat per day over an extended period, what is medically termed a *nonresponder*. In other words, some people could eat all the fat they wanted and nothing would happen to their cholesterol levels.

Writing about this lipid hypothesis linking diet and cholesterol, Ancel Keys from the University of Minnesota wrote:

There are good reasons for the current great interest in the effects of the diet on the blood lipids. It is now generally agreed that there is an important relationship between the concentration of certain lipid fractions in the blood and the development of atherosclerosis and the coronary heart disease it produces. The outstanding characteristic of atherosclerosis is the presence of lipid deposits, mainly cholesterol, in the walls of the arteries. And both in man and animals the most obvious factor that affects the blood lipids is the diet.[40]

It took decades before people understood that Anitschkow and indeed de Langen were far ahead of their times. As noted cardiologist Steinberg wrote about the lipid hypothesis in 2013:

The main problem was that he was too far ahead of his time. Anitschkow was born in 1885 and wrote his classic paper in 1913. Yet the validity of the lipid hypothesis did not become generally accepted until 1984 . . . We who have followed in Anitschkow's footsteps salute him on this hundredth anniversary of his breakthrough paper.[41]

A decade ago, patients were told that the level of LDL (bad) cholesterol in their blood should be less than 130 mg/dL if you were moderate risk (two or more risk factors for heart disease that create a 10 to 20 percent chance of having a heart attack in the next ten years) and less than 100 mg/dL if you were high risk (history of heart disease or diabetes). There was also a view that when it came to LDL cholesterol, the lower, the better—if LDL levels are pushed down to sixty or so with statin medications, the risk of heart attack and other cardiovascular events falls further than if LDL levels are pushed down to just ninety or so. For very high-risk patients, following recent heart or vascular surgery, the target was 70 mg/dL. For HDL (good) cholesterol, the target was a minimum of 40 mg/dL.

However, the problem with using specific levels of cholesterol as targets was the lack of evidence, and truth be told, many in the medical profession were simply using guesstimates—there was a lack of solid science behind cholesterol levels. Of course, companies that manufactured drugs loved these recommendations. When has a lack of scientific precision hindered commercial production or trade?

When it came to HDL, it was felt the higher, the better. However, there is a problem with this good/bad theory of cholesterol. In theory, it sounds good because the HDL acts to remove cholesterol from specialized cells called macrophages, which helps to prevent the buildup of cholesterol in our blood vessels. HDL also has antioxidant and anti-inflammatory properties. Moreover, when HDL is damaged, it can actually damage blood vessels. We saw this in the previous chapter, that the stress response is also a double-edged sword. Research now shows that emotional stress actually raises cholesterol levels.[42]

Why does this happen? The plasma membranes of all cells contain glycosphingolipids (a rather complicated chemical name, but essentially a type of fat and a sugar combined) and protein receptors organized in lipid rafts. These may as well be called life rafts as, without cholesterol, life would be impossible, since cholesterol is heavily involved in signaling (cellular communication), maintenance of cellular membranes, and surfactant stabilization (surfactants are oils that prevent the alveolar air sacs of the lungs from sticking together when babies exhale)—all essential when there is increased activity and readiness to fight or flee when an animal is under threat.

This good/bad cholesterol hypothesis actually came from a study that investigated the effects of vitamin B_3, niacin, on cholesterol levels.[43] It was found that niacin lowered LDL cholesterol (which we already knew was bad) and raised the HDL cholesterol (which, by proxy, had to be good, right?). But this theory hit a snag when drugs called CETP-inhibitors were studied (remember how wild mice lacked CETP and therefore had more good cholesterol). When torcetrapib—

a CETP inhibitor drug produced by the drug company Pfizer—was tested along with a statin, it ended up causing deaths, as it increased blood pressure that led to strokes or heart attacks, showing that for cholesterol in humans, there is a thin line between good and evil.

Previously, physicians were expected to treat patients to bring cholesterol levels below 100mg/dL, with the ideal being 70mg/dL. Now all targets have been removed, as the science simply didn't stack up. The committee instead focused on using cholesterol-lowering medications, statins, to reduce LDL—without a particular target.[44] Statins were classified by the committee as high intensity (shown to lower LDL by at least 50 percent) or moderate intensity (lower LDL by more than 30 percent but less than 50 percent).[45] Anyone aged twenty-one to seventy-five with cardiovascular disease, LDL greater than 190 mg/dL, or aged forty to seventy-five with diabetes is recommended to take a high-intensity statin, much to the relief of drug companies that make such medications. Indeed, many cardiologists even believe that statins should be introduced into drinking water as a public health measure. However, statins are not without risk, and the main adverse effects include muscle pain or damage, liver damage, and even memory loss. Beyond that, there is no uniformly accepted treatment (yet) for statin-induced muscle disease.

One of the problems with how the cholesterol story has evolved is that the science was ignored long enough that it now appears dubious. Previously, everyone was monitoring cholesterol levels only to be now told that they don't really matter. Truth be told, most people just want to know the practical things, like whether they can eat eggs or bacon. From the public's perspective, the messages are confusing, as evidenced by a fifty-year-old patient of mine who was worried because his father had a heart attack at age fifty-three: "Doctor, regarding eggs, are they good or bad? For years, we've been told that eggs are bad, but now I'm told that we can eat eggs without worrying about cholesterol."

Let's look at a single egg. According to the US Department of Agriculture, one large egg contains 186 milligrams of cholesterol.[46] The main problem when it comes to eggs is not the eggs but their accompaniments, typically processed meats like bacon and ham, which are high in trans fats. Processed foods contain these inherently unhealthy trans fats as well. If you are healthy, it is perfectly safe to have an egg a day. According to the Mayo Clinic information sheet, it is better to avoid eating more than three hundred milligrams of cholesterol per day, and if you have diabetes or heart disease, then you are better off limiting your cholesterol intake to under two hundred milligrams per day.[47]

In response to a paper published in the *New England Journal of Medicine* titled "Normal Plasma Cholesterol in Man Who Eats 25 Eggs a Day," Ancel Keys, who is considered the father of the diet-heart theories, wrote a letter stating:

> Dietary cholesterol has an important effect on the cholesterol level in the blood of chickens and rabbits, but many controlled experiments have shown that dietary cholesterol has a limited effect in humans. Adding cholesterol to a cholesterol-free diet raises the blood level in humans, but when added to an unrestricted diet, it has a minimal effect.[48]

In Anitschkow's original experiment, he fed his rabbits cholesterol when their usual diet was cholesterol free. Therein lay the problem with his study—the design was elegant, but the deductions were misleading. What developed were fat deposits, different from human plaques. After all, the human liver produces its own cholesterol, which is essential for optimal functioning of the body's membranes and hormones. Therefore, if our diets are fairly constant daily and consist of varied food groups, adding cholesterol has a minimal effect.

Fat cells are rather unbound by conventions or shame. The cell numbers are constant at birth, but the cells themselves can move, collide, and expand greatly. By contrast, cholesterol can be unlimited, but it is defined by type and location. Cholesterol is essential for maintaining cell membranes, and indeed there is evidence that as fat cells, the adipocytes, increase in size, they need their own cholesterol factory to maintain the structural integrity of their cell membranes. So it follows that obesity increases cholesterol production partly to stoke this supply.

However, high cholesterol levels may result in a reduction in the volume of gray matter in the brain. The gray matter is essentially the processing unit of the brain, as it contains nerve cells and their branches; the white matter contains the axons, the insulated wires that interconnect regions of the brain. Studies have shown that gray matter is reduced by high cholesterol levels, even in people without dementia.[49] Dr. Joseph I. Friedman, from the Icahn School of Medicine at Mount Sinai in New York, and colleagues studied brain scans of patients who had no symptoms but did have known cardiovascular risk factors—they found that high cholesterol reduced total brain volume, metabolism, and decreased brain coherence.[50] Again, fat guts, skinny brains. However, there was hope—lifestyle measures, such as aerobic exercise (both bipedal and endurance), were able to reverse these changes if diagnosed early.

The Skinny Gene

"Why don't French women get fat?" has been debated both in medical conferences and in social situations. In her book *French Women Don't Get Fat*, Mireille Guiliano talks about French attitudes toward food, and many others have also studied the "French paradox."[51] While medical researchers searched for genetic clues, there were none, except for possibly lower homocysteine levels (increased blood homocysteine and low folate is associated with heart disease).

Inhabitants of Toulouse in France have some of the lowest levels of homocysteine in the world. The MTHFR gene that is associated with both homocysteine and folate metabolism is implicated here. The French eat plenty of folate-rich vegetables, eat smaller portions (French food labels contain warnings regarding snacking between meals), consume very little fast food, do more exercise (cycling in the countryside or walking up stairs to old apartments), take coffee without milk, drink red wine, and eat small portions of cheese (cheeses like Brie actually stimulate cholecystokinin, which makes one feel full faster). Therefore, the French fondness for eating croissants ultimately ends up having minimal effect.

There is also a gene that makes people naturally skinny, and it is possible that the prevalence of this gene for slenderness is higher in thin populations that are known to eat a lot of saturated fat. Recent clinical studies have shown that the effects of saturated fats on obesity can be influenced by variations in a gene called APOA2.[52] If you possess the TT or TC variant of the APOA2 gene, there is no increased risk of high obesity with a diet high in saturated fat, but if you have a CC variant of the same gene, you had better stay away from fried and baked foods.

As to plasma levels of homocysteine, increased BMI and gut fatness may be associated with increased plasma homocysteine, which is also implicated in decreased brain function (it causes Alzheimer's dementia) and insulin resistance. The latter causes diabetes, which results from excessive sugar intake.

We know from studies that doubling or even tripling saturated fat in a constant diet does not increase cholesterol levels in the blood; however, we now also know that increasing sugars, especially fructose, promotes a rise in cholesterol levels. Therefore, it is especially important to reduce refined or added sugars that are found in many processed foods. Sugar is considered the new fat because carbohydrates such as refined sugars induce leptin resistance, which, as we saw earlier, makes one become both more overweight and hungrier.

If there were any doubts about the effects of sugar being worse than fat, they were extinguished when a study that looked at the effect of glucose levels on the higher end of the normal range in people in their sixties showed that high normal blood glucose (borderline blood-sugar levels that almost reach diabetic levels) is associated with decreasing brain volumes and dementia.[53] Again, it's skinny brains, fat guts, even if the real cause is sugar. Fructose is often implicated, because many processed sweets contain high-fructose corn syrup. Both fructose and glucose increase the production of triglyceride fats, which are implicated in arterial disease and diabetes. Notably, fructose also impairs removal of these fats, while glucose does not.[54] This important difference is why, in a direct comparison, fructose induces more fat production than glucose.

One of the other concerns with the extreme restriction of cholesterol is that cholesterol plays a biological role in maintaining plasma membranes that mediate transport of neurotransmitters and helps the development of more synapses between neurons. More recently, evidence shows that cholesterol plays a major role in the neurotransmitter serotonin, a chemical known to influence stress response and mood, as we saw in the previous chapter. Low serum cholesterol can cause lower cholesterol in the brain and affects the serotonin reuptake transporter (SERT). Studies have shown that serotonergic neurotransmission is strongly connected to behaviors such as violence and suicide. Beatrice Golomb, associate professor of medicine at the University of California, San Diego and her team have spent more than a decade researching cholesterol-lowering statins and mood changes. In a survey of 843 patients on statins, Golomb reports that nearly two-thirds (65 percent) of the 843 respondents mentioned increased anxiety or irritability, and 32 percent reported an increase in depressive symptoms.[55] Another study by Golomb recently noted that men and women responded differently to statins—as their scientific paper notes: "Statins generally decreased aggression in men; and generally increased aggression in women."[56]

And studies have confirmed that people on low-fat diets generally exhibited more non-ritualized aggression involving physical contact. To simplify: significant correlation has been found between lowered cholesterol levels and violent behavior. And, as to the risk of suicide, an increase in the rate of violent suicide and violent suicide attempts was found in people following drug therapy with statins to reduce cholesterol.

From an evolutionary perspective, there were reasons to be lean and angry rather than fat and happy, as life was dangerous and man was exposed to many predators. As primitive humans consumed more food and performed more physical activity, they had larger brains. When fat and cholesterol stores were low due to starvation, the increased violence and aggression helped men undertake riskier activities such as hunting. Therefore, in some ways, cholesterol-containing food shortage acted as an alarm, neurologically mediated by serotonin levels that made men fight for and over their food. As John Naish reported in the *Daily Mail*, "The association between statins and aggression has been known for more than ten years, thanks to studies by US and Italian researchers (though this is not mentioned on the NHS Choices webpage on statin side effects)."[57]

Some cardiologists may advocate statins for every adult, but it is worth considering the dangers of cholesterol-lowering drugs and statin-addled brains. If you have a genetic tendency for high cholesterol, sure, statins may help; if not, healthier eating and exercise may be the way. The fact is that atherosclerotic plaques actually begin forming in teenage years, which makes educating children the key for future generations. Human wellness may not be intrinsic, but it is something that can be both earned and learned.

Conclusion

Stories about weight loss, body shaping, and fatness are everywhere in the media. But a whole cohort of fat-abstinence warriors may be fighting the wrong battle, as they carefully avoid disturbing the sugar-coated elephant in the room. There is corpulence and there is cholesterol—both have evolutionary stories, and there is a lot we can learn. But, ultimately, it is clear that we are simply consuming too many calories. There's more to food than guilt. A delicately grilled steak with some fancy artichoke sauce is actually okay, even accompanied by some ciabatta bread smothered with butter. All these various diets being promoted, like carb cycling and Paleo, merely induce guilt.

Ancient Homo erectus ate more meat than Homo sapiens, closer to the Paleo diet, and were more athletic, but guess what. These Paleo eaters ended up skinny but also extinct. If agriculture was all bad, it would not have ensured our longevity as a species. From an evolutionary point of view, there is economic gene theory that basically says an overweight person was more likely to be slower and therefore at greater risk of death from predators. And because the higher the weight, the smaller the brain, smarts weren't likely to have been around to help the situation. Recent studies have shown that every calorie you avoid is worth about thirty seconds of more life, so here's the real question: Are you prepared to give up a piece of cake to live another day?

If we want to learn from our past, moderation is the key. Aristotle once said, "It is better to rise from life as from a banquet—neither thirsty nor drunken."[58] In modern times, *enough* seems to be the hardest word.

Reader Rx: Family Fun

Maintaining childhood ideal body weight (BMI) helps reduce the chance of being overweight in adulthood, so make sure children reduce sugar and exercise regularly. Activities that can help are high-intensity exercises two to three times a week, ideally a combination of running, squats, jumps, and climbs. Adults might like to go to the gym, but to give the whole family a good workout, try setting up an obstacle course. Use chairs as hurdles, open the flaps of boxes to create a tunnel to crawl through, add in some jumping jacks and squats, and maybe even climb your fence. You could time each family member to see who's fastest or try to beat your personal-best times.

Another great exercise option to maintain body weight is starting a hip-hop dance team, as that provides the elements of muscular resistance, leg activity, movement variations, and endurance training.

Key Points

1. Fat cell numbers are constant throughout life.
2. Overweight children have a high likelihood of being overweight adults, so early education is key.
3. There is an inverse relationship between body fat and brain size—fat guts lead to skinny brains, and vice versa.
4. Increased BMI and abdominal fat may be associated with increased plasma homocysteine, which increases the risk of dementia and diabetes.
5. Eating a lot of cholesterol makes no difference if the diet is constant and unrestricted.

6. Omega-3 to omega-6 ratios are important—the higher the omega-3, the less the risk of heart disease and diabetes, as well as a reduction in Alzheimer's disease and rheumatoid arthritis rates, and larger brain sizes.

7. Trans fats—unsaturated fats found in margarine, fried foods, and processed fast foods—are especially bad. High sugar intake makes people both hungrier and fatter.

5

The Pigment Genes: The Myth of Race

Dermocracy
I'm saying "dermocracy," I'm saying equality
World's not saying fraternity—it doesn't talk
Not epidermis nor dermis nor genes
separate us, scientific truths remain unspoken
I'm saying skincare, I'm saying beauty
Brown doesn't say it's beautiful—it doesn't talk…
I'm saying science, I'm seeing emotion
Skin doesn't choose partners—it doesn't talk
But we see skin color when we long for somebody's
presence, whether it's black truth or a white lie

—Sharad P. Paul

In the summer of 1942, my grandfather, who was the first ethnic Indian in British India to head a church, visited the United States. My grandfather, a Lutheran pastor, hailed from Andhra Pradesh, the Telugu-speaking southern state in India and, typical of people from southern India, was quite dark skinned.

As my grandfather prepared for his first voyage to the big, boisterous, and bountiful land of America, he received an astonishing request from his gracious hosts—would he mind wearing a turban, so he could be distinguished from African Americans (referred to as negroes in those days)? What this turban was supposed to do was immediately differentiate my grandfather as being a more acceptable black man, something that would grant him safe passage while traveling in southern America. Given that people don't normally wear turbans in that part of India (unlike the Sikhs in Punjab), he had to buy a kitschy ceremonial turban, a sort of glittering gold turban that one might find in a costume store or at a gaudy Bollywood wedding. In all the excitement at being invited to America, this strange request was easily complied with, and this story and image was relegated to family folklore.

Due to my work in medicine and research mostly being to do with skin, I've always found this story interesting. Skin pigmentation can change after childhood and at a fundamental level due to stress on the body, either due to hormones (natural or due to pregnancy or oral contraceptives), environment (sun exposure), medications (some antibiotics like tetracyclines, for example), or even emotional stress. It has been estimated that around five million Americans, mostly women, seek help for skin pigmentation problems annually.[1]

Skin remains mysterious because as an organ, it is both unique and diverse. Any other organ can hide mediocrity behind layers of, well, skin. If a liver or a kidney is not up to par, you might never know unless you were to have a medical test or examination. I've often said skin wears its health like a badge for all to see—everything is unashamedly exposed.

The Evolution of Skin Pigment

Charles Darwin noted that humans had less color variation than animals:

The colour of the face differs much more widely in the various kinds of monkeys than it does in the races of man . . . we have some slight evidence that the tints of the different races were acquired at a period subsequent to the removal of the hair, which must have occurred at a very early period in the history of man.[2]

It is amazing that a single pigment, melanin, is responsible for all different skin colors of mankind—stripes on animals and all human skin colors are caused by varying levels of this pigment. Often appearing as just a speck of black on skin, melanomas, tumors of our melanin-producing cells, can be lethal skin cancers. Every hour one person dies of melanoma in America. Why do creatures have melanin anyway?

In a previous chapter, we discussed sea squirts, of brain-digesting fame. The sea squirt takes us back to a primitive earth where creatures rebelled against the domination of the sun and predation by other creatures. In ascidians like sea squirts, any offending parasite or fungus is rapidly isolated and sequestered in a capsule made of pigment and blood cells, leading to pigment-filled "scars." Guess what the pigment is? Melanin. It has the uncanny ability to appear and change creatures' appearances all the way through evolution. Melanin is the ultimate antioxidant. When the body is under threat and mitochondrial activity increases, more reactive oxygen species (ROS) are generated as by-products. These are what we sometimes term *free radicals*. Melanin is a scavenger of reactive oxygen species and vigorously defends cells or tissues from the toxic effects of free radicals. Like a Lilliputian prince of blackness, melanin is feverishly busy, constantly plotting molecular war or holding biochemical deliberations to avert biological battles. More recently, studies on fungi have shown that fungal melanin pigments have high antioxidant activity indicating that melanin is almost omnipresent. When it comes to skin the role of melanin is to protect us from environmental toxins such as sunlight.

In order to understand the evolution of skin pigment, we must first take a look at the history of the various theories that have arisen over time. Sadly, many of the theories speculate on varying values for different ethnicities, supporting racism. It was a long and winding road, but eventually science advanced enough to explain skin pigment in terms of biology: the tale of two vitamins that we'll discuss in this chapter.

History of Theories

The fifteenth and sixteenth centuries were the age of exploration, when European nations like Spain, Portugal, England, and France sent ships in search of new frontiers and fortunes. They also found exotic peoples. Unable to understand the cause of black skin, Jean Riolan the Younger, a famous Parisian anatomist, actually dissected the skin of a black "Aethiopian" subject and noted that the skin had two layers, similar to his own. Riolan called the upper layer, which was black, petite peau (horny layer), and the lower layer peau or cuire (dermis), which he noted was "white as snow."

With the assistance of a microscope, the Italian physician and biologist Marcello Malpighi discovered that the dermis and the stratum corneum (horny upper layer of epidermis) is colorless in both black and white skin, and concluded that the blackness in Africans must originate not in the skin but in the underlying mucus (what he called the *rete mucosum*). Unfortunately, while Malpighi was an original thinker, he sought a divine explanation to explain a physiological fact, theorizing that all men were probably white to begin with and that sinners ended up turning black due to their underlying mucus changing color. Utilizing a derivation of the Hebrew word *Ham* (which meant "heat" or "dark"), the prevailing teaching from Genesis 9, where Noah cursed the descendants of his son Ham to a life of slavery, was that this was an explanation for black skin. This theory prevailed as late as less than a century ago, when in 1930, C. G. Seligman wrote: "Apart from relatively late Semitic influence . . . the civilizations of Africa are the civilizations of the Hamites, its history is the record of these peoples and of their interaction with the two other African stocks, the Negro and the Bushmen."[3] However, contemporary thinking did not support Malpighi's anatomical theory of black skin, holding instead that black people were a different species of man—of course, sans souls—an extension of the Malpighi religious theory.[4]

Claude-Nicolas Le Cat, who was born in 1700 (six years after Malpighi died) and ended up the chief physician at the Hôtel-Dieu, the leading hospital in Rouen, France, came up with a revolutionary new theory in which he introduced the concept of a black substance, ethiops (hence the word "Ethiopian"). He surmised that all creatures contained this ethiops to a varying degree and that, the greater the degree of ethiops present, the blacker the person appeared. He also believed in a remarkably advanced theory for those times: that this ethiops must be contained in a specific type of bodily cell (meaning that Le Cat came pretty close to describing the concept of melanin and the melanocyte).

Le Cat's theory was similar to Malpighi's in one aspect—Le Cat also believed that it was the *rete mucosum* below the skin that determined the blackness of a person, and that the ethiops was perhaps contained in nerve endings. Le Cat had spent considerable time studying other animal tissues using a microscope. Seiche, or the cuttlefish, was one of his favorites and where he had first noted black pigment cells.

Thus, Le Cat can be considered the first person to rebut prevailing theories about the origin of skin color in humans. Those were times when some men like Giovanni Morgagni of Padua, a professor of anatomical pathology, believed that, as some black men developed the odd white patch on their skin, all black men were originally white, while others like Bernardus Siegfried Albinus and Giovanni

Domenico Sanctorini were certain that only bile could influence skin color—too much sun darkened the bile, which in turn made a person turn black. In 1741, Pierre Barrère in France wrote that negro bile was black and that is why those men were black. Claude-Nicolas Le Cat himself had a student named Jean Charles Grossard who speculated that it was perhaps the lymph of black men that was black and not their bile, but on conducting autopsies of lymphatic systems, he was surprised to find that black men and white men had lymph of the same color. It would take another two decades for Barrère to be proven wrong by Le Cat, whose theories British scientists of the time dismissed as "wild hypotheses," even if the *Gentlemen's Magazine* in 1753 recommended that Le Cat was someone who "ought to be universally read."[5] If we were to paraphrase Le Cat's early microscopic observations of the pigmented cell, they would read something like this: Melanocytes are cells containing melanin (ethiops); these are scattered throughout the epidermis but don't appear (irrespective of race) in the dermis. Epidermis and dermis are separated by a wall-like basement membrane, through which nerves cannot penetrate.

Ultimately, men like Malpighi and Le Cat were inquisitors who mounted an assault on existing theories and eventually showed that blackness could be involuntary, changeable according to the power of the sun, a means of animal cells acquiring the necessary enzymes and organelles, while the genes remained unmindful of newer postures or societal inclinations.

In 1823, Karl Friedrich Heusinger wrote a treatise on the origins of skin pigment in which he described his belief in opposing phenomena occurring inside each animal—center versus periphery, gut versus skin, and digestion versus breathing.[6] In his line of thinking, fuel was transported from the center to the periphery, and his conclusion was that carbon, derived from modified blood pigment, was deposited in the skin of all dark-skinned people. That's what made people have different colors.

A Modern Perspective of Epidermal Biology

We know Heusinger was wrong. The estimated mass of all pigment cells within our body is only around 1.5 grams, and most of this weight is made up by the melanocytes within the dermis. That's how small and ridiculous any feeling of racial superiority or inferiority is. Each melanocyte serves thirty-six keratinocytes, the outermost cells of skin. These pigment granules are then stored as melanosomes, and they spread out to cause tanning or freckling. The mistake we humans make is to confuse "expression of melanin" with color. Let's stop to acknowledge the energetic but minuscule melanin. Chemically speaking, melanin is an indolic polymer, a chain-like chemical compound that colors all animals; its blackness is due to the fact that it absorbs virtually all the visible spectrum, including radiation with low quantal energy—effectively, it's our very own cellular black hole.

Many current theories on skin, especially color, still tend to be racially biased. For example, many scientists previously suggested that white skin was more resistant to cold weather, although groups like the Inuit are both dark and well-adjusted to cold climes.

The rather inconvenient truth is that a lot of wealth was created in the years of slavery, when people were considered inferior just because of their skin color. Rich-poor theories are common in equity markets and economics. Therefore, understanding skin color for what it is—as mere biological pigment rather than human currency—can be extremely dangerous in the eyes of some people, for apportioning science and reason could destabilize entire systems of racial profiling and slavery.

Looking at Evolution through a Modern Lens

Humans and their closest living relatives, apes like chimpanzees and bonobos, were separated from their common ancestor around six million years ago, and with this severance came the differentiation into many species of humans or apes. This common ancestor was covered with dark hair and had light skin underneath. Around four million years later, or two million years ago, Homo erectus migrated out of Africa.

By now, this ancestor had a larger brain and more developed hand skills, but this brought with it certain problems. The body had to work harder to keep the brain cool (just as a computer needs a cooling fan) as physical activity and the use of hand tools increased. Although Homo erectus was not the first hominid to walk upright, he walked faster and migrated farther than other hominids, which also required cooling. To cool, he needed to sweat. To sweat properly, he required many sweat glands and a naked body. Aboriginal people—such as indigenous Australians or the Negritos who inhabit the Andaman Islands in India or the Philippines—have particularly high concentrations of sweat glands when compared to people unacclimatized to hot weather.

Apes, like chimpanzees, have black hair but light pinkish skin. As man evolved from apes, he lost the thick hair and emerged rather naked. This evolution into a naked ape necessitated a darkening of the epidermis to protect against UV damage. Skin cancers, wrinkling, and signs of aging typically spring to mind as the worst effects of UV damage. But issues like cancer or beauty are not as important from an evolutionary point of view; in all its wisdom, Nature knows that beauty doesn't last, but a species has to. The scientific explanation for the darkening of skin of our ancestors in Africa is that the sun causes photolysis, the destruction of folic acid (folate), a metabolite essential to preventing birth defects. Therefore, to preserve folic acid, and thereby the species' reproductive ability, skin evolved to become dark.

How does skin darkening—that is, increased melanin production— protect against UV damage? As a general rule, for solar radiation to produce biochemical damage, it needs to be absorbed. Melanin acts as an optical and chemical filter that reduces penetration of all UV wavelengths into subepidermal tissues. As an optical filter, it works through a scattering effect. This is made apparent by the fact that there are very few instances of folic acid deficiency in Africa, even when nutrition is relatively poor, pointing to highly melanized skin protecting against UV-induced folic acid damage.

It is no coincidence that neural tube defects, such as spina bifida and anencephaly, which are both caused by a deficit in folic acid, are far less common in the tropics, among dark-skinned people, than they are in the more temperate climates. It is also no coincidence that countries in Asia and Africa have larger populations when compared to Western countries, even with their poorer living standards and the fact that less healthcare is available during pregnancy, because reproductive issues are not as prevalent due to folic acid issues. When I graduated from medical school in India twenty-five years ago, medical doctors were not trained to routinely advocate folic acid for women planning to conceive, whereas it was already routine in Western countries, due to the much higher risk of neural tube defects.

Sunlight destroys folic acid, but it produces vitamin D, which the body needs in order to absorb calcium. Therefore the darker skinned you are, the higher your inherent folic acid levels, but correspondingly you end up with a reduced capacity to absorb vitamin D.

As the first modern humans migrated out of Africa into Europe one hundred thousand years ago, their skin lightened to allow more sun penetration to facilitate the production of vitamin D, because of the lower annual sunshine hours than in Africa. In colder, polar climates, it was even more important to produce enough vitamin D, as the sun was absent for long periods. But the lack of sun created its own problems. When dark-skinned people arrived in Europe, many developed rickets due to vitamin D deficiency, as dark skin was not transparent enough to absorb vitamin D easily.

Rickets does not only cause skeletal problems and bone deformities, but also infertility. This was a double whammy, both from a sexual selection and a natural selection point of view. Deformed individuals were less likely to be chosen as mates, and infertility ultimately bred them out. Skin, therefore, lightened to enable enough vitamin D production. There were good reasons for dark skin in Africa, but in European climes, it just did not make sense.

In dark skin that evolved in Africa, vitamin D exists in the form of vitamin D3, a precursor to vitamin D. This is the beauty of evolution's anticipatory intelligence. As skin gradually became dark in Africa over millions of years, the body could foretell a shortage of vitamin D that would occur due to the darkness of skin and produced high levels of preformed vitamin D.

Later, as white-skinned people migrated east from Europe, reached the Indian subcontinent, and ventured farther south into Asia, to more tropical climates, the skin again darkened to preserve folic acid. However, this darkening came after an initial period of lightening in Europe and therefore happened over thousands of years, as recently as four thousand to ten thousand years ago. Therefore, the body did not have time to hoard pre-vitamin D, as this darkening of skin was an *adaptive response* to preserve folic acid under the tropical sun, not an *evolutionary response* as had occurred in Africa. Therefore, Asians, especially those from the Indian subcontinent, have very low vitamin D levels.

To confirm this evolutionary theory, Martine Luxwolda studied vitamin D levels in African populations, especially in locations where early man originated and where the population was still on a traditional diet. Although she knew she would find high values, it was a surprise that the values were quite so high. Luxwolda says:

The present study indicates a mean 25(OH)D concentration of 115 nmol/l, as based on traditionally living populations with sun exposure habits that might be comparable to our African ancestors before the out-of-Africa diaspora.[7]

In their study of the "traditional people" in Tanzania, Luxwolda and her team found that this population had 115 nmol per liter (nmol/l) of vitamin D (more specifically, serum 25-hydroxyvitamin D) on average compared to the 30–60 nmol/l that Westerners had. In contrast, virtually all Indian subcontinental folk are vitamin D deficient. And because vitamin D helps muscle strength and injury recovery, the more inherent vitamin D, the better natural athletic prowess. This is why Africans and African Americans excel in athletics and may explain why India, with over a billion people, has never won even one Olympic track-and-field medal!

Thus, while the original dark color of skin in Africa was evolutionary (to preserve folic acid), once early humans had lost much of their body hair, other dark skin colors that formed were adaptive, depending on their environment. Quoting Charles Darwin again, in *The Descent of Man*:

> Of all the differences between the races of man, the colour of the skin is the most conspicuous and one of the best marked. It was formerly thought that differences of this kind could be accounted for by long exposure to different climates; but Pallas first showed that this is not tenable, and he has since been followed by almost all anthropologists. This view has been rejected chiefly because the distribution of the variously coloured races, most of whom have long inhabited their present homes, does not coincide with corresponding differences of climate.[8]

One of the discrepancies with the evolutionary theories based on the sun as a double-edged sword when it comes to vitamin D and folic acid is that we would expect the Inuit people to be lighter skinned than the Scandinavians, but they are darker skinned. This is where diet played a part in the adaptive response.

The Inuit diet is extremely rich in vitamin D due to consumption of salmon and oily fish. The European diet, in contrast, was cereal based, and so vitamin D-deficient. Over time, European skin had to adapt and become lighter to easily absorb vitamin D, whereas Inuit skin did not: cod liver oil, for example, has around 1,200 IU of vitamin D per tablespoon, and salmon has around 300 IU per ounce. If you compare that with European diets, cereals (if unfortified) contain no vitamin D and cheese only has around 4 IU per ounce. The Baltic countries—Latvia, Lithuania, and Estonia—have among the palest-skinned people in Europe because early settlers found that the warmer climates allowed them to farm grain, whereas neighboring countries like Norway and Iceland ate salmon, whales, and sharks and so had higher vitamin D levels. In my TEDx Talk, I pointed out that this was the scientific explanation behind Miss Norway having a better tan than Miss Estonia at a Miss World pageant (of course all in the interest of scientific research!).

Diet also can explain the caste system in India. The upper class Brahmins are vegetarians and therefore eat a largely cereal- and dairy-based diet. People who eat fish, such as fishermen, who were considered lower castes, had higher vitamin D levels, and over centuries, the skin of the upper castes lightened to try and absorb more vitamin D, a process that takes several centuries.

While hominids appeared 2.4 million years ago, descendants of modern man left Africa only one hundred thousand years ago. However, evolutionary responses take much longer. This is why African people in Luxwolda's study had higher vitamin D levels than Europeans even though they did not avoid sun or stay indoors like modern Asians. The evolutionary clock runs much slower than that.

So the emergence of different skin colors was essentially a tale of two vitamins—folic acid and vitamin D. We now know why skin color changed and what causes the different shades: melanin. But what were the genes that mediated this? Genes control the entire flow of hormones, vitamins, and enzymes.

There is an important skin color gene called SLC24A5, which was a major factor in color change between African and European populations. SLC24A5 is essentially a transporter (specialized proteins that facilitate transport of certain substances across cell membranes) that, in humans, is encoded by the corresponding SLC24A5 gene. While researchers are unsure how this actually regulates skin color, it seems to have something to do with the movement of calcium into cells, and we can now see the link between vitamin D, calcium, and sunlight. The SLC24A5 gene comes in two variants, dark and light. People with two dark versions (DD) are black, and people with two light versions (LL) are white—for example, people with DD would have been more likely to develop rickets when compared to those with LL versions of the SLC24A5 gene. Of course you could have combined versions and end up brown skinned.

Fish like sticklebacks often change color when they move from freshwater rivers, estuaries, and saltwater as a form of camouflage. Such changes are mediated by another gene called KITLG. It transpires that humans with two copies of the African form of the KITLG gene have darker skin color, when compared to people with one or two copies of the new KITLG variant that is common in Europe. This makes the KITLG gene one of the key regulators of skin color adaptation in both fish and humans. The change in color is regulated by the same gene in different animals, from the lowly stickleback to modern humans. This is the real "dermocracy" of skin color. What it tells us is that evolution and skin color are not merely words we encounter in a book or museum; they are glimpses into the story of our natural origins.

When nature selected these two vitamins to do battle, it perhaps forgot to reconcile with ignorant human minds—the evolutionary call was a duty, and when the order came to propagate a species, skin responded. After all, biology has no bias; humans do.

Understanding Calcium

Vitamin D is a curiosity, an aberration—it simply doesn't belong to the vitamin family. For a start, vitamins are not supposed to be produced by our bodies. As we noted, vitamin D is produced by our skin on sun exposure. I first became interested in calcium as I studied the importance of vitamin D in our health and the evolution of skin color.

When we search for life on other planets, we first look for signs of water as evidence of the land being inhabitable. It is widely accepted that the origins of life lay in underwater vents around 3.9 billion years ago. At that time, the ocean was acidic and filled with positively charged protons, while the deep sea vents spewed out bitter alkaline fluid, which was rich in negatively charged hydroxide ions—effectively like a battery that could power the chemical reactions needed to sustain life. My interest was piqued when I found that creatures underwater like starfish and sea squirts have vitamin D receptors. If humans produce vitamin D from sunlight, why did primitive creatures from the depths of the ocean even need vitamin D receptors? It turns out that this is to do with calcium metabolism.

In general, most cells have calcium concentrations around 100nM—or 100 billionths of a meter—and most structures within the cells such as mitochondria contain around 1nM. Creatures that have exoskeletons (shells) or endoskeletons (bones or cartilages) need calcium to maintain those structures. Seawater contains a much higher calcium concentration than freshwater. As creatures moved out of salt water with its 10 nM calcium concentration into freshwater (calcium 0.5–1 nM), their cells had already become adapted to functioning within a specific calcium concentration. The cells didn't know how to manage their calcium, especially as the creatures began migrating to different environments. A daringly inventive biochemical plan was hatched by evolution—why not create a calcium regulator?

Enter vitamin D. In my view, it is perhaps the most ancient *hormone.* If your vitamin D level is low, it can affect your health, as calcium leeches out of your bones to try and maintain your cellular calcium, but without a regulator, the task becomes impossible. Vitamin D deficiency leads to calcium deficiency, and when we have low calcium levels, our bodies increase levels of two hormones, parathormone and calcitriol, that increase absorption of calcium from the intestines. This leads to more calcium inside our cells (intracellular calcium). High intracellular calcium levels lead to higher blood pressure and cellular fat. This finding—that low dietary calcium raises intracellular calcium—has been called the "calcium paradox," and it has been suggested that it may also play a part in the development of arteriosclerosis, Alzheimer's disease, diabetes, and muscular dystrophy. With a high vegetarian population and dark skin, India is now seeing an increase in heart disease, diabetes, and arterial disease, even in people who maintain healthy diets.

As an ancient and evolutionary hormone, vitamin D is unique. Survival of the fittest is an imperfect idea, and many organs and, indeed, chemicals become expendable. Present in both plants and animals, vitamin D manages to achieve evolutionary indispensability. Without vitamin D, cells lose their mojo, calcium metabolism lacks equilibrium, and humans cannot grow properly. Vitamin D, the chemical, is however an odd fellow, as plants and animals have different versions—vitamin D2, found in plants and better known as ergocalciferol, and vitamin D3, found in animal tissues and referred to as cholecalciferol. Perhaps the reason we call this vitamin D is because it is easier than saying cholecalciferol, but something being difficult to pronounce does not mean it lacks purpose.

Skin Pigment in the Modern Era

Today, everyone seems to have some discomfort with their skin pigmentation. In Australia and New Zealand, people wish they were a bit more "olive," so they'd get less skin cancer. In Asia, as a skin doctor, I am constantly asked by people if I can make them a potion or lotion for lighter skin—a legacy of caste and colonialism. We've just studied the origins of skin color, but what makes our bodies produce melanin?

Remarkably, it is the level of melanin that is responsible for producing all the shades of skin color known to mankind—not just every skin tone, but also animal coat and bird feather colors too, including the inky-black plumage of the crow or the brown of a sparrow.

The word *melanin* derives from the Greek word *melanos* ("dark"), and its first use is usually attributed to the Swedish chemist Jöns Jacob Berzelius, born in Linköping, Sweden, in 1779. Berzelius lost both his parents when he was young but managed to complete school and trained to become a medical doctor, even though his life's work ended up being experimental chemistry. An ardent defender of the need for research to separate fact from opinion, Berzelius once wrote, "The habit of an opinion often leads to the complete conviction of its truth, it hides the weaker parts of it, and makes us incapable of accepting the proofs against it."[9]

The interesting thing about melanin is that it is responsible for the color of the substantia nigra (literally "black substance") of the brain, where dopaminergic neurons (cells that regulate dopamine) are found. While dopaminergic neurons only make up 5 percent of the substantia nigra, they are highly influential in our responses to reward and anxiety. Injecting dopamine into the hypothalamus of the human brain can decrease our appetite and food intake. Remember when we discussed dopamine as a pleasure particle?

If these dopamine-rich neurons are deficient, it leads to Parkinson's disease, which is a well-known cause of tremors, and the incidence

of this disease is on the rise. If there is an overactivity of these dopaminergic neurons in the substantia nigra, you can develop schizophrenia, and that leads to delusions and bizarre behavior. However, as a cutaneous oncologist, I also know that the risk of having a lethal melanoma is higher when one has Parkinson's disease (up to seven times higher), and lower when one has schizophrenia. Melanin may be the unexpected defender of our cells, the knight in chess, but the problem with this tiny speck of pigment is that every time we scientists come up with a new theory to understand it, it tends to reveal a new move.

All cellular systems, whether human or not, are powered by ATP (which stands for *adenosine triphosphate*, a complex molecule). Energy is produced from the ATP molecule by a reaction that removes one of the phosphate-oxygen groups, leaving behind adenosine diphosphate (ADP), which as the name indicates, contains two phosphates. This ADP then gets recycled in the mitochondria, which function as the batteries that power all living cells. Just as monetary currencies keep our societies functioning, this "hooking and unhooking that last phosphate [on ATP] is what keeps the whole world operating."[10] All biological processes such as plant photosynthesis, human respiration, and yeast fermentation utilize ATP.

Cells also contain organelles called *lysosomes*, which are essentially enzyme-rich structures. We now know that melanosomes, the granules that contain melanin, are nothing but lysosomes that secrete pigment instead of enzymes, and this pigment colors our hair and skin.

So it stands to reason that melanin may be the ultimate antioxidant but it ends up a double-edged sword. Melanin is increased in situations of stress and inflammation, and as we discussed in the previous chapter on stress, the same cellular changes are initiated in emotional stress, physical injury, and aging, any of which can lead to increased pigmentation of skin.

Studies have shown that smokers are more than twice as likely to develop wrinkles compared to nonsmokers. When I was in Europe recently, I was astounded as to how many young women were smoking heavily indoors. Smoking alone does more damage to your skin than you can repair with cosmetics. Drinking a lot of alcohol also dehydrates skin and so causes more wrinkling. The more stressed your cellular systems (or you) are, the worse your skin will look. One cannot have bad health and good skin.

One of the ways in which UV radiation damages deeper connective tissue is by causing reactive oxygen species (ROS). ROS, which we discussed earlier, include superoxide anion, peroxide, and singlet oxygen. Another system is related to hydrogen peroxide. In human skin and human keratinocytes, hydrogen peroxide levels are increased within fifteen minutes of UV irradiation and continue to accumulate for approximately sixty minutes after UV exposure. UV damage also degrades collagen and reduces procollagen gene expression, which, of course, makes you look older.

In his poem "Skin," Philip Larkin calls skin "that unfakeable surface."[11] Our skin cannot be fooled. If we break every rule about good food, we bully our bodies with alcohol and cigarettes, and we cook our skin endlessly under the sun, how can we blame others when things don't end up looking good on the outside?

Vitamin D and Folic Acid in Modern Diets

As I have said, in my medical practice, I have noted that almost all my patients of the Indian subcontinental skin type, irrespective of where they were born, seem to lack adequate vitamin D levels. In adults, vitamin D deficiency can not only lead to brittle bones and teeth, but also affect general health. It affects children too, though. For instance, while breast-feeding is good for a baby, if the mother is vitamin D deficient, it can lead to the baby becoming deficient and other serious problems. Many infant formulas are actually fortified with vitamin D for this reason.

Indian/Asian skin types are more prone to vitamin D deficiency because of sun avoidance (to avoid tanning or skin darkening) and dietary factors (large vegetarian populations), and the inefficiency of dark skin in absorbing vitamin D.

Traditional wisdom was that calcium intake is important for bone development, and women in India and Asia were prescribed calcium supplements. However, large medical studies (such as the Harvard nurses' study) have shown that vitamin D intake is more important than high calcium intake for preventing hip fractures, because without a calcium regulator, there is no point consuming calcium. Hip bone strength correlates with the risk of osteoporosis—bone scans to assess how brittle your bones are routinely measure "hip fracture scores."

The evolutionary battles between folic acid and melanin and vitamin D and melanin had some unintended consequences in that different skin types are predisposed to certain conditions. We now know that as humans migrated out of Africa, so did bears. Polar bears, therefore, are descendants of brown bears. But as these bears reached the North Pole, their fur was bleached by the harsh Arctic sun—the closer one gets to a pole, the stronger the sun's UV rays. But the South Pole is worse. Antarctica is a snowy mountain, while the Arctic is essentially a massive lump of floating ice. Snow reflects 20 to 100 percent of all wavelengths depending on how pure the snow is, whereas water only reflects 6 to 12 percent of visible light and half that amount of UVB radiation. However, the polar bear diet was so rich in salmon and fish oils that its skin did not need to lighten. Diets high in salmon result in high vitamin D levels and led to the benefits of fish oils being noted around fifty years ago, when studies of the Inuit population's low heart-disease rate were done. Researchers found that they had a diet rich in long-chain fatty acids. This finding later led to the industry behind fish oil capsules and supplements. But does fish oil work the same as eating fish?

A research team from Italy set out to study the benefits of fish oil consumption as opposed to simply consuming fish.For six weeks, volunteers were given either 100 grams per day of salmon or fish oil capsules (one to three per day). The findings showed that fatty acids are more effectively absorbed and incorporated into our plasma fats when we eat fish than when take them as capsules. [12] William S. Harris and others repeated a similar study that again showed that, when it comes to nutrients, eating them in their natural form is best.[13] This is because, when it is made into a capsule form, many of the anti-inflammatory properties of fish oil are lost.

There is often some confusion between vitamin D and omega-3 fatty acids. Fish oil contains both, so people often assume they are the same and have similar properties. In the absence of a calcium regulator, low vitamin D levels increase heart disease rates. We know that fish oil has been shown to be beneficial for the heart, hence the confusion between the two.

In the chapter "Skinny Brains, Fat Guts," I spoke about fish oils and the importance of omega-3 fish oils. Essential fatty acids are linoleic acid (LA), an omega-6 fatty acid, and alpha-linolenic acid (ALA), an omega-3 fatty acid. The former produces arachidonic acid, which is implicated in inflammatory reactions; many anti-inflammatory drugs inhibit this metabolism. ALA, however, can be converted to eicosapentaenoic acid (EPA), which has known cardio-protective abilities. Flaxseed oil, often touted for its omega-3 content, has only about one-sixth the efficacy of fish oil when it comes to making EPA. Because EPA and DHA are derived from ALA, and linseed oil and walnut oil also contain ALA, there were reports that those products were as good as fish oil. However, that has not turned out to be the case, because humans cannot convert ALA into DHA efficiently.

But increasingly, research has focused on the two most beneficial omega-3 fatty acids—EPA and DHA. Scientists have found that these have slightly different benefits and cannot simply be lumped together under one category. EPA, for example, strangles the production of arachidonic acid, reducing inflammatory effects, both to do with arteries and arthritis. DHA, however, does not inhibit arachidonic acid and does not have much effect on cellular inflammation. However, when EPA enters the brain, it gets oxidized, so DHA is better for brain development and an important factor in nerve function. Both EPA and DHA don't alter cholesterol levels much, and they both reduce harmful triglyceride levels.

We now know that DHA is beneficial for babies in the womb and in early childhood for development of the brain and nervous system. DHA is produced in the uterus in the last trimester of pregnancy, to support rapid growth and brain development. The baby cannot produce DHA, getting this fatty acid from the mother. Indeed, preterm infants have lower DHA levels as the ability to convert ALA to DHA improves when a baby is full term.

In 1992, Alan Lucas and colleagues at the MRC Dunn Nutrition Research Unit at Cambridge, published in *The Lancet* that breast-fed babies had a higher IQ than formula-fed babies, and this is also thought to be due to the DHA content of breast milk.[14] Another study of twenty-nine women found that children whose mothers had taken DHA supplements during pregnancy had significantly better problem-solving skills at nine months of age. DHA supplements during pregnancy are now routinely recommended.[15] Interestingly, in this study, DHA improved problem solving but not memory—the latter seems to be helped by EPA.

In fact, the 2010 US Department of Health and Human Services dietary guidelines recommend that women who are pregnant or breast-feeding "consume eight to twelve ounces of seafood per week from a variety of seafood types."[16] This is equivalent to around 300 to 900 milligrams of EPA and DHA per day.

EPA has cardiac benefits. Its neurological benefits come later in life, when it has been shown to have some benefits against memory loss and dementia. A Harvard Health publication noted: "In large amounts (several grams a day), fish oil has been shown to nudge various cardiac risk factors ('good' HDL cholesterol, triglycerides, blood pressure) in the right direction. Smaller amounts (a gram a day) (may) work against irregular heart rhythms—particularly atrial fibrillation."[17] However, overall, evidence to date suggests that DHA is more efficient in decreasing blood pressure, heart rate, and platelet aggregation compared to EPA.[18]

We know that vitamin D and omega-3 fatty acids are linked but different entities. Some fish, like salmon and cod, are especially rich in both. Cod liver oil has around 1200 IU of vitamin D per tablespoon, and salmon has around 300 IU per ounce. When it comes to omega-3 content, wild coho salmon also contains 900 milligrams per five-ounce serving, and Australian barramundi has 833 milligrams per five-ounce serving, followed by swordfish at 600 milligrams per five-ounce serving. And studies now confirm that omega-3 activates vitamin D, and this may be one mechanism of its protective effect on the heart. A study in South Korea concluded:

Omega-3 supplementation has been shown to reduce the risk of cardiovascular disease. In addition, the biologically active metabolite 1,25(OH)D has anti-inflammatory, antiproliferative, and antifibrotic effects in both the endothelial and smooth muscle cells of the vascular wall. Therefore, based on our present study, the cardio-protective effect of omega-3 fatty acids can be partially explained by vitamin D activation.[19]

Increasingly, the science behind calcium and fish oils point to the origins of life underwater. It is as if this truth is too big for our cells to hide. The sobering thought is that evolution is a dictatorial force—it gives us no choice in our creation, only in the possibility of change. Our freedom is, at best, partial.

Beyond Pigment: Melanin

Josefina López, in her play *Unconquered Spirits*, writes a story of God as a cookie maker—sometimes cookies turn out burned (black), sometimes undercooked (white), and sometimes just right (brown).[20]

Perhaps God would have smiled and confessed that he didn't own an oven, because he had already created the sun. "And I only needed one ingredient to create all the different colors of humankind," God would have said, "and the same substance makes tigers have stripes and leopards have spots."

Melanin is an ancient antioxidant. We know that cells that renew themselves constantly, like those of the cervix or lips, have a higher risk of cancer. Melanocytes, melanin-producing cells, renew themselves periodically. Hairs, which contain abundant melanin, are constantly undergoing growth (anagen), cessation (catagen), and rest (telogen) phases—in fact if we were to pluck hairs from someone's scalp, one hair might be in the anagen phase, and another in the telogen phase of the hair cycle.

Melanocytes in the hair bulb produce offspring at each hair cycle and may also be implicated in melanoma. At a more surface level, the melanocytes in the epidermis, the top layer of skin, are produced in response to ultraviolet radiation, for example, after sunburns. In the case of the hair bulb, an area where stem cells congregate, genetic dysfunction could lead to aberrant growth of cells. Where UV damage is concerned, DNA damage accumulates in melanocytes until the DNA repair army is overcome.

Melanocytes make up only 5 to 10 percent of the cells in the basal layer of the epidermis. Although their size can vary, a single melanocyte is typically seven micrometers—or seven millionths of a meter—in length. This tiny cell is capable of many actions—sadly, murder is one of them.

In my skin cancer practice, I offer a free full-body screening service. As many people cannot afford to see a dermatologist, plastic surgeon, or private specialist and given our high incidence of skin cancer Down Under, I see over seven thousand patients annually at no fee, which to date makes for over one hundred thousand free skin examinations. I've seen prime ministers and ministers, doctors and lawyers, cooks and clerks.

José Andrés Puerta, the Spanish-American chef who pioneered small-plate dining in America, once said, "I believe no chef becomes what he becomes without having many people influence him."[21] Medical practice can be like that.

One of my most memorable patients was Mike. Over the years, I treated Mike for many skin cancers—basal cell, squamous cell, and a melanoma on his scalp. Every year, on my birthday, Saint Patrick's Day, he would turn up with a bottle of wine. "That's for saving my life," he would say. Truth be told, I am not sure I saved his life, although being told such is a delicious boost to every doctor's vanity.

That he lasted so long must have been Mike's Irish luck. Melanomas are unpredictable; we see patients with thin tumors that seem harmless die from them, and we see thick tumors that are expected to kill become dormant. It's like a melanoma doesn't want a perfect beginning, or end, for that matter. Perhaps this ambiguity is all part of a grand plan—a diagnosis of melanoma forces us to seize the moment and make the best of life without knowing what's going to happen next.

Several years ago, *Sunday*, a New Zealand current affairs show, decided to make a story of my multifaceted life and they interviewed Mike. "What do you want to say about Dr. Paul?" Mike was asked.

"He saved my life," Mike said proudly, turning toward me.

Mike had survived removal of his neck lymph nodes after a melanoma, radiotherapy after removal of an aggressive squamous cell cancer, and a multitude of skin cancers. He wore his scars proudly, even if some of them I would have rather refashioned than claimed ownership of.

"How can a little speck kill anyone?" Mike asked me when I first diagnosed his condition and warned him about the prognosis.

"I know, it seems far-fetched even to doctors," I replied, "but that dark pigment is melanin, and it is a tumor of melanocytes, the cells that contain melanin."

"If a melanocyte contains melanin, where does the melanocyte come from?" Mike asked.

"That is a rather complex question," I said, giving him a brief explanation about antioxidants being double-edged swords. "We'll be here all day if I go into that. Tell me how your move into the rest home went."

"Retirement village, *not* rest home," Mike corrected me.

Mike and his wife had recently moved into a retirement village. "It isn't for me," he would say, "but if something happened to me, I want Betty to be looked after. I don't want our daughter to be burdened with looking after us in our old age."

Typical Mike—always worrying about others. A classic worrywart. We would have long conversations about Ireland: his prowess with the Irish flute, and the band that he had formed in his retirement village. And we discussed daughters. Mike had one. I had one. We were both doting dads. Fathers and daughters can be complicated . . . the genetic trigonometry of love.

My bookstore/café, Baci Lounge, in Auckland, used to have live music on some nights. I promised Mike I would get his band over— they could play a few songs and enjoy supper in our café afterward.

That Saint Patrick's Day, Mike came to see me as usual with a bottle of wine. He looked worried. "My daughter is going to lose her house," he said. She had been the victim of a fraudster who had targeted parents of children at the private school where Mike's granddaughter went and had used her house as security for an investment that turned out to be a scam. Mike was devastated. He suddenly looked old. The stress response hastens aging just as it worsens medical conditions.

That was the first Saint Patrick's Day we hardly spoke. Not that I can recall, anyway—it seemed we both were afraid to break the silence. A few months later, Mike's melanoma returned. He had been cancer free for over ten years and suddenly, amid all this emotional strife, a harbinger. I was called to see him at a rest home where he had been admitted, as Betty was unable to manage him at home as he had deteriorated almost overnight. He looked drained. The thing about cancer is that it not only lays low the adversary, but it also ravages the habitat they share. Mike's melanoma had taken over his mind and memory. All of our conversations and laughs were now gone.

I could only watch as his wife and daughter tried to explain to Mike who I was. He didn't know me. He didn't even know who they were. There was some kind of a conclusion here, an inescapable truth that heralded the end of our friendship. He seemed to nod as I said hello. But this could have been my imagination. His hands trembled. The Mike I knew was no more. I walked out of that place hastily, tears clouding my vision. It took me a while to find my car, and when I finally located it, I sat there alone for a while doing nothing. I sobbed. The entire visit seemed strangely incomplete.

I never saw Mike again. I never got to organize the dinner for his band. Another reminder that the best strategy is this—when you think you must do something for someone, someday—just do it.

Wherever Mike is, I know he'll be in a place called Ireland where his band will always play on St. Patrick's Day. My birthday.

As a doctor, I am blessed to partake in this daily narrative from my clients—patient histories, family stories and reminiscences. One reason I also trained in family medicine after initially training in plastic surgery is the rough narratives of patients, chopped up into carefully controlled time slots of medical appointments. Good stories. Great stories. Sad stories. In the end, all patient notes and investigation results end up like good novels—unpredictable to the very end. If we could all see the last page of the story of our lives, would we change how we live our lives? Ultimately, we end up as characters in these stories, and that is where our immortality lies.

Skin Cancer

Evolution does not care about skin cancer—it only considers matters of reproduction important, and because skin cancers generally occur in older age groups, when the reproductive peak is past, evolution has not made any changes that help us avoid skin cancer.

Australia is interesting from a skin evolution point of view because of the high UV index, plentiful sunshine hours, and large European populations—that weren't designed to live in such high-UV conditions—especially from Celtic countries like Scotland and Ireland. For many decades, Australia had an openly stated "white Australia" immigration policy that encouraged people of European descent to migrate there preferentially over other races. But white Australians never adapted to suit the land—their ancestors were people whose skin had lightened in Europe due to the scarcity of sun, which explains why Australia has one of the highest incidences of skin cancer in the world. On the other hand, among the Australian aboriginal population, which emerged out of Africa sixty-five thousand years ago, there are virtually no skin cancers. Geography matters, just as genes do. As I detailed in my book *Skin, A Biography,* having two copies of the MC1R gene makes you a redhead. Less than 2 percent of the world's population is ginger, but Celtic countries have many more. Scotland boasts the highest percentage of natural redheads at 13 percent and Ireland comes in second with 10 percent. In these countries, 40 percent carry the gene, even if only a quarter of these carry two copies. People with two MC1R genes freckle, cannot tan well, and end up with many more mutations when exposed to sunlight. It's because their skin adapted to live in countries where UV radiation is infrequent.

UV radiation comes in three different forms—UVA (implicated in aging and melanoma), UVB (that causes sunburns and other skin cancers), and UVC (that can cause cataracts, even if most does not reach the ground surface).

Our DNA is double stranded, like two parallel, wavy ribbons of nucleic acids. These nucleic acids are usually in a particular sequence A-T-G-C (Adenine-Thymine-Guanine-Cytosine)—a sort of yin and yang of biological compounds necessary for life. When skin is exposed to UV radiation, photons in the radiation cause damage to the DNA by altering its nucleic acid sequences into dimers—that is, it leads to the formation of A-T A-T dimers, abnormal yang-yang, yin-yin nucleic acid sequences. This is biological treason. If these sequences are not repaired, the abnormal DNA divides abnormally, leading to the production of skin cancer cells later on. Therefore, the body mobilizes certain enzymes to bring this sequence back to normal.

In dark skin that has an abundance of melanin, not too many dimers are created (because the large melanosome shields the nucleus where the DNA is stored) and the bodily enzymes are more than capable of repairing the damage. In redheaded, white-skinned people, for example, due to the lack of a large melanosome sitting above and shielding the nucleus, the DNA sustains severe damage, meaning several pairs of dimers are created. The body mobilizes enzymes, but the enzyme stores are often not enough to repair the damage properly, leading to a higher risk of skin cancer later on.

I often use diabetes as an analogy when teaching my students the DNA theory. Everyone is born with a supply of insulin in the pancreas. Some people are born with a genetic deficiency, and this leads to type 1 diabetes in childhood; this is the rarer form of diabetes, and these people need insulin injections their entire lives. Most people who develop type 2 diabetes do so because they have eaten too much over time, and this overindulgence makes them run out of insulin stores in middle age. Therefore, they need to take pills that increase insulin production or improve tissue uptake; some of these people end up on insulin injections. With our fondness for carbohydrates and overeating, type 2 diabetes is becoming all too common these days.

Similarly, some people are born with a deficiency of the enzymes that repair skin damage from UV radiation. This genetic deficiency is called xeroderma pigmentosum. These people develop a multitude of skin cancers. White-skinned people do have these enzymes. But excessive exposure to the sun, overuse of tanning beds, or a severe sunburn damages the skin until repair systems can no longer cope, which then leads to skin cancer. In Queensland, Australia, after running around all day at the beach, it was almost a rite of passage for young teenagers to run a hot bath and peel skin off each other's backs because they had sustained blistering sunburns! No wonder, then, that Queensland has one of the highest incidences of melanoma in the world—nearly eighty incidences per one hundred thousand people. Fortunately, this practice is less prevalent these days due to increasing awareness of skin cancer.

To summarize, the reason our skin darkens when exposed to UV radiation is because tanning is inherently a defense mechanism, as melanin is a sunscreen. A sunscreen with an SPF of 2 would allow you to double your sun exposure. Nobuhiko Kobayashi and James J. Nordlund, among others, studied the sun-protection factor of melanin and found that melanin has an SPF of 2 to 4. In other words, melanin will absorb 25 percent to 75 percent of UV rays (usually around 50 percent in brown skin).

But there is still a lot of confusion regarding tanning and sun protection, even among experts. Given that my team and I research and manufacture sunscreens, I was asked by my friend Rachel McAdam, who is the scientific communications and education manager for skincare company La Roche-Posay, a division of L'Oréal Australia, whether or not it was true that only UVB radiation produced vitamin D.

This is only partly true. Studies show that in short bursts, UVA and UVB do the same thing, but on longer exposure, say after nine minutes, UVA can degrade vitamin D. If you were letting in UVB rays, you would still have an increased risk of non-melanoma skin cancers, especially squamous and basal cell cancers. If you let in UVB rays selectively, then the production of vitamin D would depend on preexisting baseline cholesterol and vitamin D levels—and not on skin type or pigmentation. So the SPF calculation then goes out the window because it is not universal in individuals.

Sunscreen science is not as straightforward as we think. However, we do know that sunscreens help prevent skin cancer by reducing sunburns, provided they are applied correctly and reapplied every few hours.

Nevertheless, many people avoid using sunscreens because they worry about vitamin D deficiency. The truth is that sunscreen makes no difference to vitamin D levels—the percentage of body surface exposed does. UVB rays have been considered a major source of vitamin D; however, most studies used latitude or time as proxies for actual measurement of UV radiation on skin and did not actually measure UVB levels. In 2011, Morten K. B. Bogh carried out experiments measuring various UV doses with skin exposure; significant UVB responses correlated with 6 percent and 12 percent body-surface exposure but became saturated at 24 percent body-surface exposure.[22] What this study revealed is that we should have around 18 percent of our body surface exposed to sunlight to get enough vitamin D—this is like having both arms exposed or both legs below the knee. Therefore, it is the body surface area exposed that matters. Sun exposure of twenty to thirty minutes twice a day is sufficient, as more exposure can degrade vitamin D.

However, people who already have high vitamin D levels are less likely to get much more vitamin D increase from sun exposure. It's the way the body regulates the regulator.

Conclusion

After my recent TEDx Talk, a lady came up and asked me about the link between vitamin D and multiple sclerosis, as her mother had low vitamin D and suffered from multiple sclerosis, and she was worried that the low vitamin D had caused the condition. She had come across this information when she searched Google. I explained that there was no evidence in the medical literature about a causal link between low vitamin D and multiple sclerosis. I've had patients ask me the same question regarding melanoma, especially as it is caused by excessive sun exposure and sunlight produces vitamin D. A fairly large study done of 872 melanoma patients over five years showed that serum levels of vitamin D were lower in stage IV melanoma when compared to early stage I melanoma.[23]

Ultimately, the reason that many disease states reveal low vitamin D levels merely confirms the fact that vitamin D levels simply reflect a healthy state: The "sunshine vitamin" may simply be a barometer of our overall health. Life evolved underwater, and for creatures that ended up on land like man, vitamin D and omega-3 are like biological memories of our origins. We know that all vitamins are useful, but what about vitamin D, an ancient hormone masquerading as a vitamin? Is this substance an evolutionary miracle? More and more, science and medicine are converging toward this grand conclusion.

The subtitle of this chapter, "The Myth of Race," comes from a TEDx Talk I was asked to deliver. I spoke about how vitamin D and folic acid shaped humanity's colors and ended the talk by saying, "if the world were truly color blind, then every human being in every corner of this world could reach their full potential, and we would finally come to understand that the myth of race has not served humanity well."

Reader Rx: Lather Up

Calculate your sun "burn time" using the chart below and use SPF accordingly to help keep your skin healthy. Dermatologists and plastic surgeons often refer to Fitzpatrick skin types, which are:

- Type I: Always burns, never tans (like the typical Irish redhead or platinum blond)
- Type II: Burns easily, tans with difficulty (usually blond and blue-eyed)
- Type III: Rarely burns, tans easily (usually brown-black hair and brown-eyed)
- Type IV: Never burns, tans well (Mediterranean, Spanish, or lighter Indian skin)
- Type V: Dark-brown skin that never burns but tans easily (darker Indian skin, some North African skin)
- Type VI: Black African skin (skin that has abundant melanin and does not burn and tans easily, although this darkening is often not visible due to the extremely dark skin tone)

From a practical point of view, knowing your Fitzpatrick skin type and UV index is very useful for safe sun exposure for skin types I to IV. Skin types V and VI almost never get sunburned so are exempt from this exercise. The chart below shows an estimated "burn time" for our skin when exposed to the sun:

Skin type I	Skin type II
Maximum time in the sun = 67 minutes / UV index	Maximum time in the sun = 100 minutes / UV index
Skin type III	**Skin type IV**
Maximum time in the sun = 200 minutes / UV index	Maximum time in the sun = 300 minutes / UV index

Now calculate your SPF: From the chart above, a person with type IV skin can have a safe sun exposure of 300 minutes/ UV index. If the UV index of your city is typically ten in summer, safe sun exposure time (without tanning) would be 300/10, so thirty minutes. If you used a sunblock of SPF 15, you could expose yourself for fifteen times the safe limit, provided the sunblock was reapplied every few hours. In general, it is better to aim for a sunscreen that has SPF 30, and remember to reapply every few hours when you are out in the sun.

After sun exposure of twenty to thirty minutes, your vitamin D absorption plateaus. So it is best to have brief sun exposure several times a day and avoid peak UV hours, approximately noon to 3:00 PM.

Key Points

1. All human beings evolved out of Africa and the concept of varying races by skin color is a myth.

2. All skin colors formed because of the competition between vitamin D and folic acid.

3. Over the last fifty thousand years, human diets also resulted in modifications to skin color, mostly due to vitamin D content of foods.

4. All skin colors are due to the pigment melanin; the more melanin you have, the better you can tan.

5. Melanin has an inherent SPF of 2 to 4. The lighter your skin, the greater your risk of skin cancer.

6. Vitamin D is our calcium regulator, and normal vitamin D levels reflect a healthy state. Taking calcium supplements or eating a high-calcium diet without correcting vitamin D levels first may increase health risks.

7. Skin is both a barrier and a reflector. Therefore, adjusting our external environment (reducing sun exposure or stopping smoking) and internal environment (stress levels) are both important.

6

THE FOOD GENES: EAT RIGHT FOR YOUR GENE TYPE

This above all: to thine own self be true,
And it must follow, as the night the day,
Thou canst not then be false to any man.

—Hamlet, William Shakespeare

Patients often ask me about food allergies or what they can (or cannot) eat to improve their skin. The reason our guts matter is because our digestive systems not only provide us with fuel to function, but they also shape our internal cellular environments. We've already discussed how the environment and genes are entwined. This may be even more pertinent when it comes to the digestive system because ancient foods may have left genetic footprints, but modern foods are often made with synthetic chemicals that may have repercussions on our wellness.

As you know by now, I am not into rigid diets—because with any regimen comes compulsion, compunction, and guilt. Having said that, humanity is physically at its heaviest in history, and with this corpulence come questions like these:

Is saturated fat bad?
How much sugar can I have?
Baked or fried potatoes?

Britain has just introduced a sugar tax. Historically, there have been salt taxes and prohibition on alcohol—while raising prices by increasing taxes on certain things can bring down consumption, the problem is that laws seek to bind, not educate. All such regulations end up doing is increasing a kind of food trafficking, whereby industries simply try to get around legislations. Food is our sustenance—it shouldn't be a platform for politics or industry; it should be a platform our bodies function well on. So let's get rid of hunger, remove guilt, get educated instead, and eat healthy.

The old adage about the way to a man's heart being through the stomach makes food a currency of love—and for humans, a recent religion. The Italians practice it with great gusto, and the French excel in culinary catechism. But certain foods do make us happy, and others may cause illness in certain people due to genetic variations in our gut metabolisms—especially when diets are not balanced. When it comes to food etiquette, genes work on the concept of good and bad, rather than polite and rude. In this chapter, we will discuss different food types and their genetic implications.

The Three S's: Salt, Sugar, and Starch

In *Revolution*, Jennifer Donnelly writes: "The more obscure our tastes, the greater the proof of our genius."[1] There's a word for the savory taste found in foods like coffee, Parmesan cheese, Marmite, mushrooms, and cured meats: umami. It's thought to be in foods due to glutamate, an amino acid needed for brain function. Monosodium glutamate (MSG), the chemical found in many processed foods, naturally has this taste, as does human breast milk.[2] From an evolutionary perspective, umami taste receptors evolved for us to sense glutamate to help our brains, while bitter taste receptors evolved to detect poisons.

I begin with salt only because salt is connected to the origins of life, in the depths of the seawater. Is life possible without salt? Possibly not; in differing doses, salt has historically been a medicine to help wounds heal and to induce vomiting. Of course, it has had wide use as a preservative. Learning our origins, saline and otherwise, and understanding the origins of our species' sustenance is important. Ultimately, we have to do this for ourselves—we owe it to our bodies.

Salt

Before the age of hunting tools, people simply ate fruits and vegetables or tried to grab small insects. Even when meat began to be eaten and made up the majority of the diet, humans' salt intake was still most likely less than 1500 milligrams per day. In fact, even today, the Yanomani Indians in Brazil, who inhabit rainforests and still retain ancient dietary patterns, consume less than 500 milligrams of sodium per day. In contrast, a single can of tomato soup can contain 880 milligrams of salt.[3]

While primitive, tool-less hominids ate very little salt, salt attained great importance with the advent of hunting, as people realized its value as a preservative. Saltiness would have, in the early stages, been an acquired taste until genes began doing their thing. But this is not the only reason salt is heavily used in processed food and artificial flavorings now. Salt in higher concentration suppresses bitter taste, which means that adding salt makes processed food less bitter and, therefore, tastier.[4] As the chemicals in our processed foods are bitter when consumed on their own, salt is added, often in alarmingly high quantities. A high salt intake has clearly been shown to increase heart disease and deaths from heart disease and strokes. In spite of the medical evidence, industry lobby groups like the Salt Institute resist restrictions on salt concentrations, suggesting that there is no statistical evidence.[5]

An experiment on chimpanzees showed that those that were raised on a high salt diet developed high blood pressure, whereas their siblings on a normal diet did not. We know that salt is irrevocably linked to kidney function—kidneys either retain or excrete salt based on the direction given by certain hormones. Further proof of the link between high salt intake and kidney disease is confirmed by the fact that any inherited diseases that end up causing kidney problems tend to increase salt absorption by the kidneys. Meta-analyses have shown that reducing salt does lower blood pressure.[6] Interestingly, even though preference for the taste of salt is not present at birth, infants between four and twenty-three months old begin to show a preference for moderately salty solutions over water, and increased salt diets in infants can also cause higher blood pressure by age seven![7]

Professor Graham MacGregor from the Wolfson Institute of Preventive Medicine and honorary consultant physician at Saint George's Hospital, London gave a lecture titled "Salt: Neptune's Poisoned Chalice" in which he stated, "Mammals are designed to live away from the sea and not eat salt."[8] Marine mammals that feed on fish consume food with a salt content similar to that of their own blood, thereby avoiding fluid retention or leakage. They don't consume added salt. He went on to say:

> Unfortunately, the Chinese five thousand years ago discovered that salt had the magic property of preserving food. Salt became of great economic, religious, and political significance, but at the cost of putting up our blood pressure; [it's also] the major cause of strokes, heart failure, and heart

attacks. We are now eating twenty to fifty times more salt than we are designed to.[9]

Again, we are consuming all this salt because it is added into our foods as a preservative or to mask bitter tastes. Preserving food may have helped it last longer, but it had unintended consequences for humans, as MacGregor's next point shows:

> Some of this salt stays in our body and puts up our blood pressure; 60 percent of the population have raised blood pressure at the age of sixty.
>
> The food industry is responsible for 80 percent of our salt intake [which is] hidden in processed foods, fast foods, etc., and they must take responsibility for the thousands of unnecessary deaths and suffering they are causing . . . for each one gram reduction in salt, approximately six thousand deaths are prevented.[10]

That's a lot of lives saved! Many packaged foods and drinks contain sodium. Nowadays, salt restriction is taken to mean less than 1600 milligrams per day. That may not seem like much, but remember, our ancestors ate less than 1500 milligrams per day. One might think this alone would be enough to inspire people to cut salt out of their diets. Yet we all know people who eat a lot of salt. My father eats the most salt of anyone in our family, and yet his blood pressure is normal at age eighty-three. Clinical studies have confirmed that the effect of sodium intake on blood pressure is influenced by variations in a gene called angiotensin-converting enzyme (ACE).[11] I decided to find out what variant of the ACE gene I had—GA and AA variants of the ACE gene increase your risk of blood pressure when you eat salt, whereas the GG variant does not. It turns out that I have the AA variant and therefore need to watch my salt intake.

ACE regulates blood pressure in response to salt intake. ACE inhibitors are well-known medications for lowering blood pressure and are used to treat kidney diseases and diabetes. However, we also now know that what variant of the ACE gene you have affects your risk of developing high blood pressure due to salt intake.

In America, the African American population has a much higher risk of high blood pressure, both due to a higher intake of processed food and genetic remnants from the slave-trading era—because slaves needed to survive the difficult trans-Atlantic voyage and brutal conditions of imprisonment while awaiting transport, it is said a slave trader used to lick a slave's face to assess his fitness for voyage—salty sweat was presumably bad, as it indicated less salt-retaining properties. This taste test was meant to identify good salt-retaining people who were hardy enough to survive the long ocean crossing. However, when these people were chosen selectively for this quality, the African American population ended up with more of these salt-retaining genes and a higher risk of high blood pressure.

I've seen a picture of a slave trader assessing his slave thus in a copper engraving by Serge Daget (circa 1725) reproduced by Morris Brown in an article on hypertension and ethnic groups.[12] This "slavery hypothesis" explains the origins of higher blood pressure risk in African Americans—people who were chosen for those salt-retaining properties ended up on the same continent, cohabiting with other slaves, and this resulted in a population with a higher concentration of salt-retaining people. That was in the days before the genome was mapped; however, since we now know that our salt metabolism is determined by our genes, this could be a valid reason why African Americans have a genetic predisposition for high blood pressure. A genetic variation of the MYH9 region on chromosome 22, which is related to kidney disease and salt retention, was found in 74 percent of African Americans and in only 4 percent of Americans of European descent.[13]

I've listed the sodium content of some foods in the chart below. You may find some results surprising.

Sodium Content of Common Foods[14]

Food sources	Serving	Sodium (mg)
Bagel, egg	4" bagel	449
Carbonated drink, root beer	1 can	48
Cereal, ready-to-eat, Kellogg's Crispix	1 cup	222
Cheese (blue), cheese (feta)	1 oz.	395, 316
Cheesecake, commercially prepared	1 piece	166
Chicken drumstick, fried with batter	1 drumstick	194
Chocolate drink with whole milk	1 cup	154
Cornmeal enriched, yellow (normal, self-rising)	1 cup	4, 1860
Crackers, plain (rye, wheat)	1 wafer	87, 64
Crustacean, Alaskan king crab	3 oz.	911
Fried egg	1 large	94
Fast food, pizza chain	1 slice	670
Fast food, burrito with meat and beans	1 sandwich	668
Fast food, cheeseburger	1 sandwich	1051
Fast food, plain hot dog	1 sandwich	670
Salmon (smoked, cooked dry heat)	3 oz.	667, 59
Grape juice, sweetened with vitamin C	1 cup	15
Ham, sliced, extra lean	2 slices	627

Kiwifruit	1 medium	2
Lamb shank, roasted	3 oz.	62
Lemon juice canned or bottled	1 cup	51
Thick chocolate milkshake	1 cup	333
Candy, KIT KAT wafer bar	1 bar (1.5 oz.)	23
Candy, M&M milk chocolate	10 pieces	4
Mollusks, oysters (raw, cooked)	6 medium	177, 354
Mollusks, scallop, fried	6 large	432
Muffin, oat bran	1 muffin	224

And, if you are wondering how much salt you need in your diet, the truth is we need very little. Our ancestors managed with 1.5 grams, and the WHO recommends that adults consume less than 5 grams (just under a teaspoon) of salt per day. These recommendations apply to all individuals, with or without high blood pressure (including pregnant and lactating women), except individuals with illnesses that specifically need sugar replacement or have interactions with sodium-lowering medications such as antidepressants.

Sugar

When we say sugar, generally people think of table sugar. That is actually sucrose, which is manufactured from sugarcane or sugar beet, depending on which part of the world you are in. Sucrose contains glucose and fructose, two simple sugars. Glucose is the body's natural sugar, as it is the body's circulating sugar and is used in metabolism and for generating energy. Fructose, or fruit sugar, is the one that gets a bad rap, as it is often the culprit in causing weight gain. The body uses the glucose to generate energy, and if the excess energy from the fructose is not burned by activity, our body creates insulin that converts the fructose into fat. Researchers blame high intake of fructose as an important causative factor in the development of metabolic syndromes—diabetes, obesity, insulin resistance, and abnormal fat profile—and have come up with a new medical term, *diabesity*.[15]

But there's more we need to understand about sugar. Firstly, glucose is essential for life. Human beings are wired to binge on highly palatable, energy-rich food as an evolutionary mechanism. This mechanism developed from a time when we weren't surrounded by food and had to make do with whatever was available, with no guarantee of a next meal. Even primitive cells use glucose. A study done on yeast cells showed that the presence of sugar increased cell cooperation[16]; that is, when sugar was low, cells cooperated and did not monopolize all the available sugar. For the first 1.5 billion years of life, creatures only had one cell and swarmed over the earth. Given that they were sharing and depleting resources, this sugar cooperation is now considered one of the reasons that cells clumped together. And once they were clumped together, different cells took on different functions—and presto, we had more complex creatures!

Secondly, although glucose is essential for life, eating sugar is *not* essential; the body is capable of producing sugars from proteins (amino acids convert to sugars) and fats (glycerol and fatty acids split away and the former can produce glucose). Many creatures cannot taste sugar at all.

Humans have taste sensors, called G protein–coupled receptors (T1Rs). In humans, T1R1 senses the umami taste, and T1R2 and T1R3 sense sweetness, both natural and artificial. Tests in mice where these sensors were knocked out showed that, without them, one cannot taste sweetness.

Because of the human fetish for sugar and sweets, our industrial societies began to manufacture artificial chemical sweeteners. It took the not-so-humble hummingbird to shed light on the evolutionary biology of such sugary tastes. Hummingbirds love sugar, but when fed artificial sweeteners—the same ones that are often found in manufactured carbonated drinks—they spat them out, the same way they do plant poisons.[17] Smart birds, as artificial sweeteners are even worse for you than sugar is. What made hummingbirds smarter than humans? Essentially hummingbirds transformed their ancient umami receptors into sweet tasters. Why? Birds descended from carnivorous dinosaurs, and as hummingbirds began eating nectar, it helped their globalization, as sweet fruits and nectar were everywhere. Today, humans have also become a global colony. And with our ability to mass-produce our nectar, we are living a hummingbird's dream but with catastrophic health consequences.

The sugar debate is full of misconceptions. Everywhere in the media, fructose gets bad press. Sure, fructose can cause more fat production when compared to glucose, but is it the fructose or the quantity we are consuming? High fructose corn syrup, the mass-produced version present in many packaged foods, has long been considered the culprit. But since taste receptors cannot differentiate fructose sources, Britain's sugar tax applies to all sugary drinks and does not exclude honey.

Essentially, several studies have tried substituting different types of sugars only to conclude that the problem lies with the amount we are consuming; we know that too much sugar can make us overweight and cause diabetes, and we know that fructose is the main sugar in our carbonated drinks, but the real issue is the amount of sugar. Many carbonated drinks contain caffeine, and when caffeine is present, manufacturers automatically increase sugar content, as caffeine dulls sugar taste receptors. The caffeine content of drinks like Coca-Cola mean that they have to be made supersweet for you to be able to taste the sweetness. We also know that the younger a person is introduced to a sugary diet, the more addictive it becomes. In young children, sugar also acts as a painkiller, and due to this analgesic effect, many medicines have been historically given with the proverbial spoonful of sugar.

In America, where high fructose corn syrup is added to many soft drinks and processed baked goods, fructose currently accounts for 10 percent of the caloric intake for US citizens, and contributes to weight gain, physical inactivity, and body fat deposition.[18]

Sadly, today, even in places where food is scarce, we manage to find high levels of sugar in carbonated drinks. Research shows that once people are used to bingeing on sugars, they become like "drug dependent rats" due to changes in the opioid-secreting parts of the brain.[19] Fats can be addictive too, but there's a key difference—opiate-like withdrawal signs occur after stopping high-sugar diets, but not high-fat diets. Also, it is the sweet taste that is largely responsible for producing addiction-like behaviors, including withdrawal syndrome, making it more difficult to wean yourself off a high-sugar diet than a high-fat one—and therein lies the problem.

As sweet taste is addictive like a drug, several papers have concluded that your preference for sweet taste is proportional to your proclivity to drink alcohol. For some reason, I thought about Ireland—not least because I was headed there for the Dalkey Book Festival, alongside Malcolm Gladwell, as I was writing this. Most of the Irish I know are skinny, but science says that their famous tendency to drink alcohol also means they've got a sweet tooth. I decided to check the statistics on obesity: Ireland's overall obesity rate is 56.8 percent (in comparison to Australia's 49 percent, Brazil's 40.6 percent, China's 18.9 percent, and Denmark's 41.7 percent), which was a surprise to me.[20] If I still had any doubts about the science, I received this invite from a tour company: "Sweet Tooth? Come to Ireland."[21] Forget Guinness, it turns out that your choice of white wine determines not only your sugar preference but also your personality type—studies show that if you prefer sweeter white wines, you are a more impulsive person, but also a more secretive or less open person, indicating that a wine tasting occasion may be useful as a dating venue, if only for the psychological profiling![22]

If you have a sugar preference gene, you won't know when to stop eating sugar or drinking wine.

And now we know our guts also function as sugar sensors, that is, glucose sensing in the brain is similar to glucose sensing in pancreatic cells. Thus, newer research suggests that people who have a particular genetic anomaly may be at a higher risk of developing a sugar addiction.[23] And this sugar-craving is to do with how we transport glucose in our intestines. We do this in two ways— one is the traditional sodium channel inside cells, and the other is a glucose transporter type 2 (GLUT2) that allows glucose to leach out of cells. Hummingbirds and humans both have these transporters. What this indicates is that the expression of this GLUT2 gene has been found in areas of the brain that make you like or dislike eating sugar.

If you possess the CT or TT variant of the GLUT2 gene, your sweet tooth can be blamed on your genes: one in five adults have these gene types. If you are one of them, it is important to keep your intake of added sugar low. The chart below lists high-sugar foods that are no good for our bodies. Remember, I mentioned how caffeinated

High-Sugar Foods[24]

Sources of high-sugar foods	Amount (g)
Cola (1 can)	36
Orange juice, commercial (1 can)	32
Caramels (40 g)	26
Milk chocolate (50 g)	26
Jellybeans (10)	20
Jam (1 Tbsp)	10
Popsicle (75 g)	10
Maple syrup (2 Tbsp)	24

fizzy drinks need to have more sugar to be palatable? It is no wonder that cola tops the list!

The WHO recommends that we derive not more than 5 percent of our calories from sugar. For an average human, with a normal BMI, that works out to about six teaspoons—or twenty-five grams—of sugar per day. One can of cola or two tablespoons of maple syrup means that you've already exceeded your daily sugar limit.

Starch

Why do some of us handle starchy foods better than others? Do our ancestral origins as hunters or farmers make any genetic difference? Researchers looked at early population groups with a high-starch diet such as European Americans and the Japanese; for low-starch eaters, they chose two rainforest hunter-gatherers, the Mbuti and Biaka, and two pastoralist groups, the Datog and Yakut. The results showed that the more starch you ate, the more amylase (the enzyme that breaks down starch) you contained in your saliva. This was evolution at its culinary finest, tinkering with genes to help us avoid indigestion. Instead of creating a version of a gene that helped break down starch, these folks had a higher number of the same gene. This is genetically what we term *copy number variation*. And interestingly, this coincided with agriculture and people setting up homes. Not only did the starch eating cause more amylase genes to appear, but people who made extra amylase were healthier and had more kids. Therefore, in some ways, man's consumption of starchy foods can be considered a step toward domestication of man himself.[25]

An interesting study that compared wolves and domesticated dogs found that three genes, AMY2B, MGAM, and SGLT1, were activated around 10,000 to 3,000 years ago, coinciding with the timeframe when dogs were first domesticated. These adaptations allowed the early ancestors of modern dogs to thrive on a diet rich in starch relative to the carnivorous diet of wolves, as wolves cannot digest starch. The authors of this study concluded that this was a "striking case of parallel evolution" during the period of early agriculture, when both dogs and men developed genes to cope with starchy diets.[26] Man's best friend ended up not just a friend in need, but a friend in feed.

Now, starches are probably the most misunderstood of foods. Many recent diets espouse the mantra "carbs are bad," but is it really that simple? Starches contain carbohydrates, which are sugars, both simple and complex. All simple sugars like glucose or fructose have the same formula C6H12O6. Glucose is the immediate source of energy for cellular respiration; fructose is the sweetest of simple sugars and called "fruit sugar," as it is found in fruits and honey. But long-chain complex sugars (starches) are different. Starches are generally classified by their ability to raise your sugar levels, and this determines their glycemic index (GI). The New Zealand Nutrition Foundation explains this nicely:

> A food's GI indicates the rate at which the carbohydrate in that food is broken down into glucose and absorbed from the gut into the blood. In high GI foods, this occurs quickly, causing your blood glucose (sugar) level to rise rapidly. In low GI foods, carbohydrate is digested slowly, resulting in a more gradual rise in blood glucose levels.[27]

Therefore, low GI foods are inherently preferable. Food preparation also has a bearing on GI, and this is where Mediterranean cooking methods shine. In Britain, they mash potatoes; in Italy, a study found that their traditional dumplings, made by mixing cooked, mashed potato with wheat flour and boiling them a second time reduced the GI index considerably.[28] While mashed potatoes have higher GI, these dumplings had lower starch availability, and this has led to the concept of "resistant starch." Therefore, potatoes are not all bad; it is often the method of cooking that matters. The *Sydney Morning Herald* newspaper ran an article "In Defense of Potatoes" which reported, "While instant mashed potato earns a high GI of 86, peeled baked Pontiacs a high GI of 93, and boiled, peeled Desirees a GI of 101, unpeeled Carisma potatoes score a low GI of 55, providing you cook them the right way—cut into 1 centimeter slices and cooked until they're still firm or al dente."[29]

Starch basically contains amylose (which makes about 20 to 30 percent of the starch) and amylopectin (70 to 80 percent)—the former is soluble, while starches like rice, with high amylopectin content, become sticky when cooked. For example, glutinous rice used in Asian cooking contains the highest amount of amylopectin and is therefore sweeter—the lower the amylose, the higher the GI index. As Professor Jennie Brand-Miller sums up: "The only whole (intact) grain food with a high GI index is low amylose rice, such as Calrose rice . . . However, some varieties of rice (basmati, a long grain fragrant rice) have intermediate GI indices because they have a higher amylose content than normal rice."[30] Rice bran, in comparison, had a very low glycemic index. When it comes to rice, the higher the amylose, the lower the GI; when it comes to potatoes, GI is related to polyphenol content—the higher the polyphenols, the lower the GI. Polyphenols are compounds that have high antioxidant properties, and in general, the more colored a vegetable is, the greater its polyphenol content. In fact, the antioxidant activity of solidly pigmented red or purple potatoes is comparable to brussels sprouts or spinach as long as the skin is consumed, and they have twice the antioxidant activity of white potatoes.

Resistant starch is another recent addition to the nutritionist's lexicon. It is basically starch that isn't fully broken down and absorbed, but rather turned into short-chain fatty acids by intestinal bacteria. Therefore, amylose that we just discussed has another benefit—since it is tightly packed, chemically speaking, it is more resistant to digestion.

This makes it not only a good source of fiber but also a prebiotic. Prebiotics are essentially carbohydrates that the body cannot break down without helpful bacteria or probiotics. Prebiotics become food for probiotics, and so they induce the growth of these good gut bacteria that are in turn needed to break down such resistant starches. Brown rice, which is high in resistant starch, has been shown to reduce both blood sugars and triglycerides. Resistant starch (RS) is a recent buzzword in consumer magazines and research but is often considered together with GI. The method of cooking a certain grain may also affect the RS content. For example, when studies were done on cassava, the most common starch consumed in Brazil, the cassava-based dessert, sago, showed significantly higher RS content when compared to the normal cassava flour.[31]

For an at-a-glance reference on GI for various common starches, see the chart below.

Glycemic Index of Rice, Pasta, and Potatoes[32]

Food Source	Approximate Glycemic Index (Glucose = 100)
Rice, white	83
Rice, brown	66
Rice, bran	19
Pasta, wheat	58
Pasta, brown rice	92
Oats, rolled	58
Barley, rolled	66
Bread, white	71
Mashed potatoes, instant	87
Red potato, hot (boiled)	89
Potato, french fries	63

Some manufacturers like Uncle Ben's "convert rice"—they make white rice from brown rice that has been soaked, steamed under pressure, then dried and milled—and end up with a very low GI, as low as 38.[33]

Glycemic index can also be affected by the acidity of the meal—hence sourdough breads, common in Mediterranean countries and Israel, have a lower Gl, as does soluble fiber. Therefore, whole grains like barley, quinoa, brown rice, and buckwheat lower the risk of diabetes, and again there is a genetic throwback to our past. In a study done on American women, the TCF7L2 gene was found to be a predictor of the likelihood of developing type 2 diabetes. People with the high-risk GT or TT variant of the gene are at greater risk of developing type 2 diabetes, so are better off consuming more whole grains.[34]

AMY1 is the gene that codes for the enzyme amylase, which as I mentioned earlier, helps us digest starch. If your ancestors consumed more starch, you are more likely to have the TT or AT variant of the AMY1 gene, in comparison to those whose ancestors consumed lower-carbohydrate (starch) diets; those people often end up with the AA variant and find it difficult to digest starch.[35] Having problems with your penne or sensitive to spaghetti? The answer may lie in your genes.

Intolerances

It can seem like the world is becoming increasingly intolerant, not only when it comes to our food. It is as though everyone these days is allergic to something. Research shows that young boys and older woman are actually more prone to allergies as compared to any other gender or age group—two-thirds of food allergies are in boys, whereas, among adults, females have the greater preponderance of food intolerances (65 percent).[36]

In January 2016, I was a guest at the Jaipur Literary Festival, the world's largest literary event, attended by over three hundred thousand people. Everywhere you looked, there were literary giants or super-stars like Margaret Atwood, Stephen Fry, Colm Tóibín, and Alexander McCall Smith. I wandered into the bookstore at the festival to check out some Indian writing from small, lesser-known presses. There was an advertisement with a quote from a book: "Love is all about guts. If you have it, you fight with the world. If you don't, you fight with your-self."[37] Our guts battling our bodies over things we love to eat—that about sums up food sensitivities.

Intolerance, whether to gluten, lactose, coffee, or something else, is increasingly the way we identify ourselves. Cafés routinely offer soy milk lattes or gluten-free cakes. Magazines and newspapers write about gastric identity. How much of this indigestion is really indis-position and how much is imaginary? Perhaps the answers lie in our heredity.

Gluten

When I followed my parents into medicine, I ended up a student of medicine at Madras University. In Madras, now Chennai, my uncle, Dr. Thambiah, was a legendary dermatologist. On one occasion, there was a visiting missionary from Wales who developed a skin rash that looked rather like herpes zoster, or shingles, but did not seem to get better with time. Because my uncle had spent time in the United Kingdom and had seen many patients with white skin, which in south India still remained a curiosity at that time, someone had brought this man to see him. My uncle took one look at the man and advised him to stop eating wheat: "Stop eating the local chappatis and rotis; you can eat the rice-based idlis and dosas." One look, one dietary recom-mendation, no potions or lotions—I'm not even sure if he mentioned a specific diagnosis or not.

Skin disorder due to gluten sensitivity was first described by Dr. Louis Duhring of the University of Pennsylvania in 1884 and was named *dermatitis herpetiformis* as the rash resembled the viral vesicles caused by herpes.[38]

According to Diana Gitig in *Scientific American*, "Gluten is the primary protein component of wheat—it is what gives breads their delicious chewy texture."[39] People's intolerance to gluten was first described nearly two thousand years ago, around 150 AD, by Aretaeus of Cappadocia, on the peninsula between Asia and Europe.

As a physician, Aretaeus embodied everything that attracted me to medicine—curiosity, critical thinking, compassionate care, and clinical meticulousness. The reality of these things are quite different in modern medicine, where business drives medical practice. If you research Aretaeus, you'll find this gentleman was the first to describe the symptoms of bipolar disorders, asthma, diabetes, and, indeed, gluten intolerance.[40] In fact, when Aretaeus's works were published in Latin in 1652, his Greek word for "abdominal," *koiliaki*, was transcribed to *celiac* and ended up as *celiac disease*, a severe form of gluten intolerance. More recently, in 1950, the Dutch pediatrician Willem Dicke noted improvement in diarrheal symptoms in children fed diets that excluded wheat, rye, and oats, and this led to a greater understanding of this condition.[41]

I've often said that diagnosis in medicine is the art of observation. It's about finding something to blame in an unimpeachable body. In some ways it has less to do with the things inexperienced students see, and everything to do with unseen confounding variables. Aretaeus was remarkably observant, as his notes distinguish between mild gluten intolerance and the full-blown autoimmune variant, celiac disease:

> The stomach being the digestive organ, labours indigestion when diarrhoea seizes the patient. If this diarrhoea does not proceed from as light cause of only one or two days' duration, and if, in addition, the patient's general system be debilitated by atrophy of the body, the Coeliac Disease of a chronic nature is formed.[42]

Celiac disease is a permanent intolerance to dietary gluten and related proteins that results in immunological damage to the proximal (food-exposed) small intestine. People with celiac disease end up with all kinds of skin and joint problems, osteoporosis, anemia, and, of course, severe intestinal problems. About 1 in 133 Americans suffer from this disease, but it is very rare in Asia/India, where rice-based diets are more common. But many people have a milder form of gluten insensitivity rather than a full autoimmune condition.

Gluten is everywhere in modern diets, it seems. As Gitig says,

> The only known cure for celiac disease is complete elimination of gluten from the diet—so no pizza, bagels, pasta, pancakes, waffles, doughnuts, cookies, soy sauce (it has wheat in it), licorice (ditto) . . . you get the idea. Even communion wafers are verboten . . . It is gluten, as well as hordein and secalin, the homologous protein components of barley and rye. So no beer or malt vinegar for celiacs either.[43]

While these are common foods and avoiding these may make you a culinary dissident, if you really have gluten intolerance, then avoiding gluten is the only real cure, as consuming gluten can make your immune system respond violently, causing multisystem dysfunction.

People with celiac disease almost certainly tend to have a genetic tendency, human leucocyte antigen (HLA) type HLA-DQ2—as noted earlier, this is very rare in South India (where rice is a staple, unlike North India, where wheat predominates), and even rarer in China or Japan. In people with this genetic variant, celiac disease is noted in 99 percent of cases. It must be noted that only 1 percent of people who feel they are intolerant to gluten will actually turn out to have celiac disease. Non-celiac gluten intolerance is often not fully accepted medically. If you don't have the full autoimmune syndrome, many doctors are skeptical and may claim that it is all in patients' minds, even if people say they feel better when they avoid wheat.

However, the medical community is finally taking notice. A recent study confirmed that these two gluten-associated disorders, gluten sensitivity and celiac disease, are different clinical entities.[44] In the former, gluten activates the innate immunity and causes abdominal symptoms; in the latter, the adaptive immune responses that stimulate your T and B cells—the specialized defender cells that are found in lymph—are activated, thereby mounting a full immune response.

Nowadays, much better genetic testing is available for you to know which condition applies to you. I usually get my friend Ahmed El-Sohemy of Nutrigenomix, a Canadian corporation that specializes in dietary genetics, to run some tests for me. Essentially, approximately 99 percent of people with celiac disease and 60 percent of those with non-celiac gluten sensitivity have the DQ2 or DQ8 risk version of HLA, compared to only 30 percent of the general population. His team tests for six variations in certain HLA genes and has developed an algorithm based on gene variants that can classify individuals based on their risk for gluten intolerance: low, medium, or high.

In places like Japan, where ancestral diets were all rice based, the disease is virtually unknown until recently, which is likely due to globalization. Because human wheat cultivation is relatively recent, only ten thousand years old, this wheat eating was perhaps something evolution thought would be a passing fad and responded in the only way it knew—by triggering genes, causing a whole new medical condition (and industry) to evolve. Gluten is now the godfather of the grain mafia. Use it in bread, and you get the nice-tasting, chewy feel. Make gluten-free pizza and it tastes like plaster or slices of cardboard. But for a few unfortunates among us, science can now confirm that this insensitivity is real, and not just cutesy malingering. Novak Djokovic, the tennis superstar, talks about his gluten intolerance in his book

Serve to Win: "I had to learn to listen to my body . . . Once I did, everything changed. You could call it magic. It felt like magic."[45]

For those who are intolerant to gluten, the chart below may be helpful in identifying risky foods.

Sources of Gluten[46]

Known gluten sources	Hidden gluten sources
Bread	Salad dressing
Pasta	Pudding
Cereal	Imitation crab
Oats*	Vegan meat substitutes
Baked goods	Potato chips
Malt	French fries
Soy sauce	Soup stock
Gravy	Chocolate and candy
Barley	Processed meat
Vinegar	Canned soup
Wheat—including rye, spelt, barley	Instant rice
Beer—barley or wheat based	Ice cream

*Pure oats do not contain gluten, so look out for cross contamination

Lactose

I gave up drinking milk, whose primary sugar is lactose, a few years ago. I seemed to be getting a peptic ulcer type of pain and decided to try giving it up. It was the right call, as I've had no abdominal discomfort since. I often joke that drinking milk as an adult is unnatural. What other adult species drinks milk from its mother, let alone someone else's mother? Colleen, a friend in Canada, told me she gave up drinking milk and her skin improved dramatically. "You are a skin guy. How come you or my dermatologist never advised me to give up milk?" she asked me. This was a decade ago, when the link between milk and adult acne was not well known. In 2005, a retrospective study asked 47,355 adult women to recall their high school diet. The study was confined to those that had sought physician assistance for acne. This large study found that acne was positively associated with the reported quantity of milk ingested—particularly skim milk.[47]

Unnatural or not, humans have drunk milk and made byproducts like cheese with it for a long time. In the 1970s, a team of archeologists led by Peter Bogucki was excavating a Stone Age site in Poland. They found a pot full of tiny holes that dated back seven thousand years. At first, they weren't sure whether these holes were due to wear and tear or were deliberately created by the potter all those years ago. Bogucki, a professor at Princeton University, had seen similar vessels used by a friend to make homemade cheese. He had almost forgotten about this find until years later, in 2011, when Mélanie Roffet-Salque from the University of Bristol began to analyze the fatty residues preserved in this clay pot and concluded that they were milk fats. It was indeed an ancient cheese maker.

Genetic analyses of human remains suggest that during the ice age, most people could not possibly digest milk, so it would have been considered toxic.[48] This is because adults, unlike children, could not produce the lactase enzyme required to break down lactose. So it seems that evolution needed to find a way to make milk digestible when people began farming cattle and experimenting with milk. These early farmers found that fermenting milk to make cheese or yogurt made it more palatable. Scientifically, this is because fermentation reduces the level of lactose. This practice first began in the Middle East around eleven thousand years ago and was later adopted in Europe. The clay pot we discussed earlier was a remnant of this era. A few thousand years later, a genetic mutation spread through

Europe—one that gave people the ability to produce lactase and drink milk throughout their adult lives. Why did this happen? What was the evolutionary advantage?

We know from DNA studies that farmers replaced hunter-gatherer folk around 7000 to 7500 years ago, especially during the period when Bogucki's pottery was made in Poland. Cattle and sheep were primarily farmed for meat. Cheese and yogurt were only seen as secondary sources of food from these animals. The bacteria used in the fermentation processes are microbes like lactobacillus that reside normally in our intestines and metabolize lactose—except in people who are lactose intolerant. Of course, as we age, we all develop different degrees of lactose intolerance—our lactase levels decline, which means the lactose from milk travels to your colon undigested, where bacteria break the sugars down and create excess gas and fluid in the process, leading to the symptoms of lactose intolerance of bloating and loose stools.

Nature watches us and makes us adapt. Just as skin color evolved due to migration of people, our changing diets triggered more genes. It is widely accepted, and biologically logical, that this genetic mutation that allowed people to become lactase persistent happened with the advent of farming, when people had regular access to milk.

Jared Diamond, a Pulitzer Prize winner and author of *Guns, Germs, and Steel*, calls agriculture "the worst mistake in the history of the human race."[49] Granted, farmers had access to more food with less work when compared to hunter-gatherers. However, Diamond feels that hunter-gatherers had "plenty of leisure time, slept a good deal, and worked less hard than their farming neighbors."[50] I thought about Diamond's comments recently, as there has been a debate in New Zealand, a predominantly farming economy, regarding a shortage of local people wanting to work on dairy farms.

Diamond may be right about the farming lifestyle—grass may indeed be greener in other occupational pastures—however, something happened in Europe all those years ago that ensured milk's future as a drink. Europe was in famine, and the sick and malnourished turned to milk in desperation. This meant that those who were lactose intolerant did not survive, leaving few who were lactose tolerant alive to pass on the gene. This ensured not only the survival of the mutation for lactose persistence, but also the passing down of these genes. Loren Cordain of Colorado State University, an authority on primitive diets, also notes these further benefits of milk: it gave humans an advantage against malaria in Africa and Southern Europe and rickets in Northern Europe—in 1952, a team led by Brian Gilmore Maegraith, who was a malaria researcher at Oxford, and later the Chair of the Liverpool School of Tropical Medicine, found that milk suppressed infections in rats infected with malaria-causing *Plasmodium berghei*— so milk may have acted as an antimalarial.[51] Malaria is a massive global problem and anything that helps with malaria resistance is of huge evolutionary significance.

Farming came to Europe with folk that migrated from Turkey and the Middle East, and many of these darker-skinned folk developed rickets, a disease that causes bone problems and infertility, as their darker skin was not able to absorb vitamin D efficiently. Milk has large amounts of calcium and small amounts of vitamin D. Because vitamin D is essentially a regulator of calcium metabolism, milk would have also helped improve fertility at that time—protection against malaria and rickets were good reasons for the milk-drinking gene to evolve in adult humans.

Milk has become a huge part of everyday life and industry. It is a prime example of how culture also shapes our genes. When I moved to New Zealand, I was astounded at how much milk people drank in this "land of milk and honey." It is routine to put a baby to sleep with a milk bottle in its mouth—a recipe for chubby babies and bad teeth.

Lactose intolerance occurs because the LCT gene found in infants gradually decreases expression (activity), and this is controlled by a

SHARAD P. PAUL, MD

DNA sequence located within a nearby gene called MCM6. When we break down lactose, it turns into glucose and galactose (another sugar with the same formula as glucose and fructose: C6H12O6). Sometimes, when people are ill and the bowel is not functioning normally, we can also temporarily become lactose intolerant. We now know the risky variants of the MCM6 gene that lead to lactose intolerance: CC or CT—if you have the TT variant, you have a low or no risk of being lactose intolerant.[52]

Because milk's inclusion in certain people's diets dates back thousands of years, today's prevalence of lactose intolerance varies by geography—in America and many parts of Western Europe, or in their descendants, where dairy was a vital component of meals, lactose intolerance rates are the lowest in the world. By contrast, East Asian nations have the highest rates of lactose intolerance.[53] When early humans first wandered around Africa, they were nomadic hunter-gatherers; farming originated later, as we discussed, in the Middle East, and was then adopted in Europe—accordingly, three out of ten Europeans, or Americans of European descent, are lactose intolerant; in contrast, eight out of ten Africans, and nine out of ten Asians are lactose intolerant. My lactose intolerance was, therefore, rooted in my family's origins in Asia, even if I was born in England. When it comes to our guts, everything, it seems, can be explained either by genes or geography.

The European Food Safety Authority looked into the lactose threshold—that is, how much lactose a person could tolerate.[54] Symptoms of lactose intolerance have been described after intake of less than 6 grams of lactose in some subjects, while some could manage twice that. The chart on the next page gives you a rough idea of the lactose content of foods.

Farming brought about a milk revolution, and with it came tolerances, and intolerances, to lactose. Adding coffee to milk may have been early attempts at culinary experimentation, but it brought with it new gene expressions. Of course, for some people like Godot, the masked detective in the Ace Attorney series, milk in coffee is blasphemy: "A single drop of milk is all it takes to destroy the pure black magic in the cup!"[55] As coffee is the most-consumed beverage in most countries in the world, behind water, it's now worth looking into our coffee genes.

Sources of Lactose and the Amount Contained in Those Foods[56]

Sources of lactose	Amount (g)
Goat's milk (1 cup)	11
Cow's milk (1 cup)	12
Chocolate milk (1 cup)	10
Buttermilk (1 cup)	9
Ice cream (½ cup)	5
Cottage cheese (½ cup)	3
Sour cream (¼ cup)	2
Parmesan cheese (50g)	<1

Coffee

It is estimated that 1.6 billion cups of coffee are consumed every day.[57] Down Under, in Australia and New Zealand, cafés are everywhere, and everyone thinks he or she is a coffee connoisseur. It is almost impossible to have a serious discussion about coffee without debating single-origin coffees, brands of espresso machines, or the best methods of roasting.

It is said that coffee originated as an energy snack—coffee beans were crushed into balls of animal fat and used for quick energy during long treks and warfare by nomadic tribes in Ethiopia around 800 AD.[58]

As early as 1699, a book called *England's Happiness Improved* declared the following as the benefits of the newfound drug that was coffee: "Moderately drunk, coffee removes vapours from the brain, occasioned by fumes of wine, or other strong liquors; eases pains in the head, prevents sour belchings, and provokes appetite."[59]

The stimulation that coffee provides, the reason for its worldwide spread, is due to its caffeine content. Perhaps it was this knowledge that spawned a modern generation of manufactured caffeinated drinks like Coca-Cola and Red Bull. Unlike milk, coffee was never a primary food source, so most of the effects on the body are related to the metabolism of caffeine and are not evolutionary, but they still have genetic implications.

Caffeine has the chemical formula $C_8H_{10}N_4O_2$, and the chemical name is trimethylxanthine. It is a plant alkaloid that occurs naturally in coffee, tea, guarana, and cola nuts. It is now considered the world's most widely used drug and has a range of effects on different bodily systems as outlined below.

Caffeine and respiration: The chemical structure of caffeine is similar to that of theophylline, a bronchodilator. Therefore, caffeine is now used in asthma treatments, cough medicine, and preventing apnea in premature babies. The influential Cochrane review found that even small amounts of caffeine improve lung function for up to four hours.[60]

Caffeine and gastrointestinal system: Although coffee consumption has been shown to reduce the frequency of liver disease, it wasn't initially clear if this was due to the caffeine or some other ingredient. But a study of patients with hepatitis C showed that caffeine reduced mortality and offered some protection from worsening infectious disease in patients already suffering from one. Coffee also shows increased glucose metabolism and improves insulin sensitivity of muscles. Studies have also shown that increased coffee consumption reduces the incidence of type 2 diabetes. However, C-peptide levels that increase when more insulin is secreted were reduced in people drinking both caffeinated and decaffeinated coffee, so some of coffee's benefits seem to be independent of caffeine dosage.

Caffeine and the musculoskeletal system: Biologically, the term *autophagy* (*phagy* means "eating" and *auto* means "oneself") is a kind of self-cannibalization that occurs in plants and animals. Components of the cytoplasm are chaperoned out by vacuoles or lysosomes—both of which engulf damaged components and recycle them. This regular maintenance process aids recovery, regeneration, and longevity of cells. This process is particularly important in muscle cells—skeletal muscles have one of the highest basal rates of autophagy when compared to other tissues, and autophagy is increased when the muscle is under stress during exercise or sport. Caffeine has been shown to have a positive impact on skeletal muscle as it aids autophagy and, therefore, allows muscles to recover faster after exercise or injury. This is why levels of caffeine are monitored in athletes by drug-monitoring agencies such as WADA (World Anti-Doping Agency).

Caffeine and the nervous system: A large cohort of men and women with Parkinson's disease were studied to understand the effects of caffeine. Caffeine reduced the risk of Parkinson's disease in men and women; however, in women, it worked better if the women had never taken hormone replacement therapy (HRT). Studies were done on caffeinated and decaffeinated drinks and showed that the effect was due to caffeine, as decaffeinated coffee did not show any benefit. Other researchers have found that coffee consumption can even decrease the risk of suicide, showing that suicides decreased by 13 percent for every cup of coffee consumed daily.[61] A review of three large cohort studies was done of over 200,000 Americans and suggested that the relative-risk of suicide was 45 percent lower among individuals who consumed 2–3 cups of coffee per day, after adjusting for smoking and other variables. There was no such benefit with decaffeinated coffee, suggesting once again that it was the caffeine that mattered.[62]

This improvement in mood after coffee isn't altogether surprising, as it is a stimulant that increases the releases of dopamine.

This look into the world of coffee made me think coffee was indeed a wonder drug. Another Cochrane Review showed that adding caffeine to painkillers, such as ibuprofen or aspirin, makes them more potent and helpful when people were suffering from migraines, postoperative pain, or after childbirth.[63]

But surely, coffee must have some drawbacks. We know that in some individuals it can cause indigestion or acid-reflux symptoms. Of course, being a stimulant, it can cause insomnia or restlessness. And with regard to diabetes, any harmful effects are not from caffeine but due to additives, like cream or sugar.

Caffeine is also structurally similar to adenosine, and this increases lactic acid buildup in germ cells, which means that, in very high doses (>200 mg/kg), it affects the seminiferous tubules of the testis and can cause infertility. In normal doses, this effect was not noted. The structural similarity of caffeine to adenosine is what leads to coffee addiction—after all, coffee is a drug and caffeine withdrawal is now a recognized disorder according to the fifth edition of the *Diagnostic and Statistical Manual of Mental Disorders* (DSM), the guide used by psychiatrists. Because caffeine resembles adenosine, caffeine molecules compete for adenosine receptors in the brain and end up taking them over.[64] Dopamine, which is more effective when adenosine is not around, ends up in higher quantities (this is how caffeine helps Parkinson's disease), and as adenosine is no longer bound to receptors and floating around the brain, it gets the adrenal glands to secrete adrenaline, another stimulant. That is why we feel a buzz after drinking a strong cup of coffee.

Over time, coffee drinkers develop a tolerance—100 milligrams of caffeine is all it takes—and then you need more and more caffeine to block a significant proportion of receptors to achieve the usual effect. It is as if, without the presence of the drug (caffeine), a brain that has gotten used to operating with an artificially inflated number of adenosine receptors cannot function effectively without them, and withdrawal symptoms like headaches, tiredness, and mood changes result. However, unlike with other drugs, the effect does not last long, and one can stop cold turkey if so desired. If a person can stay off coffee for seven to twelve days, the nervous system gets reset to normal and he or she will no longer be addicted.

Overall, the benefits of coffee and moderate doses of caffeine seem wide and varied. My main medical practice is in the field of skin cancer. In cases of many soft tissue tumors and lymphomas, caffeine has even been shown to potentiate the effects of various chemotherapy drugs and is now a well-known treatment.

But some people simply cannot tolerate coffee; they develop palpitations or sometimes nausea and dizziness after consuming it. This is due to our body's mechanisms of detoxifying caffeine. Many early medicines were plant based, and the body needed to express CYP1A2 genes to detoxify these drugs. CYP1A2 is a relatively young gene, and studies of migratory patterns of early humans show that this evolved in response to dietary patterns such as the consumption of coffee.

In humans and mice, there exists a family of cytochrome P450 (CYP) genes, a large scientific superfamily that contains over a hundred protein-coding genes. These cytochrome P450 proteins catalyze many reactions involved in drug metabolism and are involved in the making of cholesterol, steroids, and other lipids. CYP1A1 and CYP1A2 are the main ones—the former seems to be an ancient gene and important for life functions, such as dealing with toxins produced by our body's own metabolism, and is not related to the metabolism of plant medicines; the latter is what breaks down caffeine.

Slow metabolizers of caffeine have a higher risk of heart attacks if they drink more than two cups of coffee per day; however, fast metabolizers actually have reduced risk of a heart attack if they have at least a cup of coffee a day. We earlier discussed how caffeine reduced risk of deaths by suicide. However, a study in Finland of middle-aged men showed increased death from heart disease by heavy coffee-drinkers.[65] Knowing your genetic type here becomes important, as when it comes to CYP1A2 and coffee, there are some interesting facts. People with the AA variant of the CYP1A2 gene are fast metabolizers, while those with the AC or CC subtypes of the gene are slow metabolizers.

A decade ago, a Canadian team led by my friend Ahmed El-Sohemy presented their findings in the *Journal of the American Medical Association* (*JAMA*) showing that the CYP1A2 gene variant may determine a person's risk of heart disease.[66]

As I mentioned earlier, I love my daily dose of coffee. But this gene business had me worried. I do get the occasional cardiac twitch after a strong cup of coffee—*maybe I have that truant coffee gene*, I thought. I decided to track down El-Sohemy and find out if my coffee gene type indicates an increased risk of heart attack. Dressed casually in a white T-shirt and jeans, Ahmed is a youthful scientist whose company specializes in nutritional genomics. He suggested that my daughter and I both be tested. While we were waiting for the results, my daughter, Natasha, teased me that I might be the one with the faulty coffee gene and could be forced either to quit coffee or end up with a faulty heart. I'm not sure which possibility worried me more.

My genetic test for the CYPA12 gene revealed a GG variant— phew! The risky ones are the GA or AA variants. My risk was not elevated, even if in general it is best to limit caffeine to 300 to 400 mg/ day. My daughter has the GA variant, meaning that, if she consumes more than 200 milligrams of caffeine a day, she could end up with heart disease. Moments after we received our test results, we went to a café—my daughter had a fruit smoothie and I had a coffee to celebrate.

In general, there are two varieties of coffee on the market produced from two different species of the *Coffea* genus: *Coffea arabica* and *Coffea canephora*, otherwise known as *Coffea robusta*. These varieties are commonly referred to as Arabica or Robusta coffees. A comparison showed that the caffeine content of an average Arabica bean was 0.8 to 1.4 percent, whereas the Robusta coffee bean had a caffeine level of 1.7 to 4.0 percent.[67] For both beans, the methods of roasting also had a bearing on caffeine levels—dark-roasted coffee has less caffeine than lighter roasts, because the roasting process reduces the caffeine content.[68]

Average Caffeine Content of Coffee Varieties[69]

Standard Coffee	Caffeine content (mg per cup)
Plunger coffee	100
Filter coffee	150
Instant coffee	65
Turkish coffee	165
Espresso or cappuccino	80 (varies in cafés up to 160 due to number of shots used)
Decaffeinated coffee	**(Café chains listed below serve 16 oz.)**
Espresso	2
Starbucks	8.6
Dunkin' Donuts	10.9
Krispy Kreme	13.9
Other caffeine sources	**(Sodas are generally 12 oz. servings)**
Coca-Cola	25–35
Diet Coke	25–47 (diet version of Coke higher)
Diet Pepsi	25–37
Red Bull	80 (similar to café coffee)

Coffee has shown antioxidant properties due to the presence of phenolic antioxidants, even if many of these benefits are lost during the roasting process. However, polyphenol derivatives, such as phenylindans, that are formed upon roasting have high antioxidant properties, meaning coffee recovers its antioxidant property to some degree. Cherry coffee of the Robusta variety, from Vietnam, had almost twice the antioxidant levels when compared with Arabica coffee.

So how much caffeine does an average cup of coffee contain? The chart on the previous page gives you an idea.

In the novel, *August 1914: The Red Wheel*, by Aleksandr Solzhenitsyn, his character Varsonofiev notes that intolerance was the first sign of an inadequate education.[70] Everywhere we go these days, people seem to be oversensitive to something—lactose, gluten, or coffee, even if sometimes these allergies are not real—so understanding our gene profile helps greatly.

Vitamins and Minerals

Vitamins are organic compounds—chemicals derived from other living matter because we cannot manufacture them. As we noted earlier, vitamin D is an imposter. Our body actually produces it, so it's not a true vitamin. Metals are generally considered trace elements, as our bodies need them in small quantities and we cannot manufacture them. Metals such as iron are usually an integral part of one or more enzymes involved in metabolic, defense, or biochemical processes. Because a deficiency of some vitamins or minerals—particularly vitamin C, vitamin A, and iron—can cause debilitating diseases, it is worth looking at the evolutionary biology and health aspects of these substances.

Vitamin C

Vitamin C deficiency has serious consequences—it has been estimated that over two million sailors died from scurvy caused by the lack of vitamin C. Famous men that circumnavigated the world noted this condition, even if they were not aware of the cause. Vasco Da Gama, who began his expedition to India in 1497, wrote on losing 100 of his 160 seamen: "Many of our men fell ill here, their feet and hands swelling, and their gums growing over their teeth so that they could not eat."[71] Later, Sir Richard Hawkins wrote: "In twenty years, since that I have used the sea, I dare take upon me to give accompt of ten thousand men consumed with scurvy" and "wished that some learned man would write of it, for it is the plague of the sea, and the spoil of mariners."[72]

In 1747, James Lind described one of the earliest double-blind trials in medicine, aboard the HMS *Salisbury*. Lind took twelve men with similar cases of scurvy—as he noted, "their cases were as similar as I could have them"—and gave half two oranges and one lemon per day; the others, he gave vinegar and seawater.[73] Lind concluded: "The most sudden and visible good effects were perceived from the use of the oranges and lemons; one of those who had taken them, being at the end of six days fit for duty."[74]

In Darwin's theory of natural selection, there is a dictum: use it or lose it. If an animal stopped using a particular organ, it eventually disappeared. Creatures that live in complete darkness have no eyes, for example. But sometimes evolution can have unintended consequences. Most primitive creatures produce their own vitamin C by converting glucose into vitamin C. Human beings, bats, and guinea pigs, however, cannot produce vitamin C. Although infants inside the uterus can produce vitamin C, this L-gulonolactone oxidase (GULO) gene gets inactivated. Since all species that have lost the capacity to synthesize vitamin C have a vitamin C–rich diet, many hypothesize that this was a result of our diet incorporating vitamin C. In other words, once apes and humans began eating fruits containing vitamin C, we may have lost our ability to synthesize the vitamin. Vitamin C may well be an example of how diet governs genomics.

We now know that low levels of vitamin C are not just related to scurvy but can also increase risk of diabetes, cancer, and cardiovascular disease. Vitamin C is an antioxidant and helps mop up free radicals. We've discussed oxidative stress previously. It appears that vitamin C compensates for increased oxidative stress that occurs in heart disease and impaired transport that occurs in diabetes. Authors of a study that looked at vitamin C supplementation among diabetics concluded: "Ascorbic acid supplementation for diabetic subjects may provide a simple means of preventing and ameliorating the complications of diabetes."[75]

The daily requirement of vitamin C for our body's needs is around 75 milligrams. The US Institute of Medicine's Food and Nutrition Board suggests the following doses of vitamin C daily:[76]

Men more than 18 years old: 90 mg
Women more than 18 years old: 75 mg
Pregnant women more than 18 years old: 85 mg
Breast-feeding women: 120 mg
Children 1–3 years old: 15 mg
Children 4–8 years old: 25 mg
Children 9–13 years old: 45 mg

Given that we now know the benefits of vitamin C and our daily requirements, what food sources could we turn to? After all, natural sources are always better than pills. The chart on the next page lists some common dietary sources of vitamin C.

But certain people do not absorb vitamin C efficiently. Studies have shown that a gene called GSTT1 is implicated in this, and your risk of vitamin C deficiency depends on the presence of an insertion or deletion (Ins or Del) variation.[77] This means that people who possess the Del variant will have at least 20 percent lower blood levels of vitamin

C and should incorporate double the daily requirements of vitamin C into their diets.

Common Foods and Their Vitamin C Content[78]

Source	Serving Size	Vitamin C (mg)
Peppers (red, yellow) raw	½ cup	101–144
Peppers (red, green) cooked	½ cup	121–132
Broccoli, raw	½ cup	42
Broccoli, cooked	½ cup	54
Guava	1 fruit	206
Kiwifruit	1 fruit	84
Tangerine or mandarin	1 fruit	22
Orange (medium sized)	1 fruit	59–83
Meat, Milk	1 cup	0

During my experiments with vitamin C, I tested my vitamin C serums on my clients. Using fluorescence spectroscopic skin scanners, we can record improvement in skin after using skin serums, especially vitamin C–based ones that help reduce skin pigmentation. We could also note the benefit in eating vitamin C in fruit form. As many dermatologists prescribe high-dose vitamin C, which is the synthetic version, I tested this and found no skin benefit. In the beginning, I thought this was an error in my analyses or scanner. But now we know that this phenomenon is well-known as *xenobiotic metabolism*—the body recognizes the synthetic version as alien. Oral vitamin C tablets may work on other internal organs, but on the skin's surface, there is no visible benefit. We only see benefits of vitamin C on skin when it is used in skin serums or consumed as food. Therefore, natural is best; as with any food source, the less processed the better.

Vitamin A

Vitamin A does not make the news as often as vitamins C and D; however, it is of ancient origin and is irrevocably linked to sunlight and vision.

Vitamin A from animal sources is *retinoid*, also called *retinol*, while plant-based vitamin A are carotenoids, such as beta-carotene. Animal sources are more readily bio available—that is, they can be used by our body instantly, without conversion. Essentially, there are three forms of animal vitamin A derivatives—retinol (the alcohol form), retinal (the aldedyde form, also called retinaldehyde), and retinoic acid (the acid form). Retinal is the precursor of the other forms of vitamin A and can be converted to retinol and vice versa. Retinoic acid is the form you often see in cosmetics to reduce wrinkles, as it helps mediate vitamin A when needed for cellular development. Increasingly, you'll see retinaldehyde in acne treatments.

Vitamin A is a heavy lifter in healthy vision. The interesting thing is that visible light corresponds to a wavelength range of 400 to 700 nanometers (nm) and a color range of violet through red. The peak absorbance is around 500 nm. Interestingly, the peak absorbance of rhodopsin, the dim light receptor, in most species is 500 nm. This is because the peak irradiance of sunlight on earth's surface is 500 nm, and moonlight is essentially reflected sunlight and therefore has the same peak irradiance. Creatures like some fish that have to see both under and out of water have many more opsins—the proteins that are receptive to vitamin A—than we humans.

In those primitive bacteria that exist even today, opsins not only acted as light gates (primitive vision) but also light pumps (primitive solar energy cells). But in higher creatures and humans, all opsins are just light receptors—for example, humans have rhodopsin within rod cells (dim light and night vision) and photopsin within cone cells (color vision).

What's vitamin A got to do with eating for our gene type? As we noted, carotenoids have to be converted into active vitamin A in the gut. Essentially, vitamin A comes in two forms: preformed (readily available) retinol from animal sources in our diet such as liver, cod liver oil, milk, and eggs; and pro-vitamin-A carotenoids from plant sources—these are beta-carotene, alpha-carotene, beta-cryptoxanthin, lycopein, lutein, and zeaxanthin—that need to be converted into active forms by the body. Preformed vitamin A retinol is about twelve times more potent—the activity or potency of vitamin A from different sources is standardized by expressing them in retinol activity equivalents (RAE): 1 RAE = 1 microgram retinol, 12 micrograms beta-carotene. This makes it easier to compare the actual vitamin A level rather than saying "milligram," for example, because of the differences between animal and plant forms of vitamin A.

We now know that there are genetic variations among people in converting vitamin A from plants. Beta-carotene mono-oxygenase 1 (BCMO1) is an enzyme that plays a key role in the conversion of beta-carotene into the active form of vitamin A and comes in variants AA, AG, and GG. The GG version holders are poor converters and therefore need to ensure they get enough preformed vitamin A from animal sources.

Sadly, while we in the West live in relatively affluent times and have access to plenty of vitamin A, the prevalence of night blindness due to vitamin A deficiency in children is almost 50 percent in south Asia and Africa simply because of the lack of food. Frighteningly, an estimated 250 million preschool children are vitamin A deficient in these regions.[79] Vitamin A deficiency is rare in Western society except in cases like anorexia nervosa or alcoholism.

The table on the next page lists some good sources of vitamin A, their RAE value, and their availability. While some foods may have higher RAE value, they may have a lower daily value percent; daily value is used by the FDA to guide consumers (for vitamin A it is 5000 IU per day).

Good Sources of Vitamin A, Their RAE Value, and Availability[80]

Source	RAE per serving	Percent of Daily Value
Egg, hard boiled	75	5
Salmon, 3 oz.	59	4
Beef liver, pan-fried, 3 oz.	6500	229
Carrots, raw, ½ cup	459	184
Broccoli, boiled, ½ cup	60	24
Mangos, raw, 1 whole	112	45
Cantaloupe, raw, ½ cup	135	54
Spinach, frozen, boiled, ½ cup	573	229
Ready-to-eat cereal fortified with vitamin A	127–149	10
Ice cream, French vanilla, 1 cup	278	20
Sweet potato, baked in skin, 1 whole	1403	561
Pumpkin pie, commercial, 1 piece	488	249
Peppers, sweet, red, raw, ½ cup	117	47

I was amazed at the content of vitamin A in pumpkin pies and sweet potatoes when compared to animal sources like eggs. It is hard to imagine Thanksgiving in America without pumpkin pie. I'm told the best way to make this vitamin A-rich pumpkin pie is in a traditional cast iron skillet. In many households, pumpkin pie spice may be a closely guarded recipe, but pumpkin pie spices have a reasonable iron content: .98 milligrams of iron per 5 grams.[81] Given the importance of iron both in industry and medicine, it is worth looking at the genetics of iron metabolism in more detail.

Iron

In *The Canterbury Tales*, in a riff about the clergy, Chaucer muses, "If gold rusts, what would iron do?"[82] Plenty, actually, as when it comes to living creatures, both microbes and men, iron is more valuable than gold. In fact, from an evolutionary or genetic point of view, the more iron a creature can accumulate, the better.

In Shakespeare's *King Lear*, egg whites were applied to raw wounds to help them heal. In the 1940s, when Arthur Schade and Leona Caroline were attempting to develop a vaccine against shigella, a diarrheal disease, they found egg whites stopped the microbes.[83] Try as they might, they could not grow microbes until they added an iron-binding compound. Take the iron out of the egg, and microbes swarmed over its defenses. This led to an understanding about the importance of iron in our immune defense systems. As a skin doctor, I often run blood tests on young patients with acne, and more often than not, a flare-up is related to iron deficiency.

Eugene Weinberg proposed that withholding iron from microbial pathogens could be a way of the body defending itself, and he called this concept *nutritional immunity*.[84] What makes iron effective when it comes to defending our biological forts? For a start, iron is an essential micronutrient for microbes, as well as their hosts, especially as it can shift between ferrous ($Fe2+$) and ferric ($Fe3+$) oxidative states, meaning it can behave both as an antioxidant and also help with electron transport. Even before Weinberg, George Cartwright and his colleagues had noted what they called *anemia of chronic infection*, which amounted to the idea that if you suffered from a long-term infection, then over time, you developed anemia.[85]

In Lewis Carroll's *Through the Looking Glass*, the Red Queen says to Alice: "Now, here, you see, it takes all the running you can do, to keep in the same place."[86] Evolution is like that—every creature competes for resources and also strives for longevity of the species. This is especially true for iron. Bacteria need it, and so do we. However, evolutionary biology forbids the use of a chemical substance exclusively for a single species. No one has the right to say, "I own this chemical substance or gene."

Iron deficiency therefore probably evolved when most of the world was malaria infested. People with low iron in their blood denied mosquito-borne bugs of vital iron they needed to survive. When iron was given to children with malaria (who had low iron) in areas where malaria was rife and medical access poor, it actually increased severe illness and death from malaria because the parasites grabbed some of the iron and recharged themselves.[87] Therefore, anemia was evolution at its defensive best—removing ammunition from weaponry lest they be stolen by microscopic marauders.

We spoke about how genes can trigger different effects based on their expression, but can people develop a genetic defect to produce too much iron? Indeed, such a disease exists, hemochromatosis, caused in most cases by a single C282Y mutation, which indicates that all this originated from one single individual. What do we know about this person? This is what we call the *founder effect*, a relatively recent gene mutation after the major migration out of Africa more common in Celtic- and Viking-descended people, but rare in Africa, and therefore originally termed the *Celtic curse*.

One theory suggests that with the advent of farming, people stopped hunting and their diets became cereal based and iron deficient, and therefore, this gene preserved more iron in the system. We noted earlier that cereal-based diets also were low in vitamin D and caused lighter skin—another Celtic curse or Celtic blessing, depending on your viewpoint.

However, as people's diets changed to once again incorporate meat with the advent of animal husbandry, this led to people developing iron overload. There is another theory proposed by Dr. Sharon Moalem that, just as malaria survival improved because of iron deficiency, the hemochromatosis gene developed as a resistance to plague, as the gene prevents *Yersinia pestis*, the offending organism, from reproducing inside of human immune cells. Indeed, the second outbreak of the plague in the fourteenth century in Europe, Asia, and Africa killed one in three humans all over the world. And we think we live in dangerous times! This extreme mortality called for desperate measures, and evolution responded in the best way it knew how—causing a genetic mutation. This theory is plausible but still unconfirmed. As Bradley Wertheim puts it in *The Atlantic*:

> Maybe C282Y is simply one of the hangers-on, a groupie following a future guitar god of the human genome: an allele with undiscovered virtuosity, currently soloing in obscurity in Mom's garage . . . But while the talent search continues, we are left wondering.[88]

Just as different creatures compete for metals like iron, even within our bodies, different organs compete for nutrients. For example, between different metallic micronutrients such as iron and manganese, it is clear that manganese competes with iron in the body—when one has low iron, one tends to have high manganese, and vice versa. This is why, when people have high manganese levels, the symptoms mimic anemia—tiredness, hair loss, and poor wound healing.

Animal and plant sources are what we call *heme* and *non-heme* iron, as the former is derived from animal hemoglobin. Non-heme iron is found in plants but is not absorbed as effectively as heme iron, and one way to increase this absorption is to consume vitamin C along with it.

We now know that there are three main genes that increase your risk of having low iron: TMPRSS6 (which codes for the protein matriptase-2, that helps to regulate iron balance); TFR2 (which helps iron enter cells); and TF (which codes for the protein transferrin that, as its name indicates, transfers iron around the body).[89] If you have variants of these three genes, and certain algorithms determine this, you will have increased iron deficiency and should consume more foods like chicken liver, boiled spinach, and the like. If consuming plant forms of iron like spinach or chickpeas, it helps to add vitamin C to your diet by eating oranges.

Conversely, given that we know variations in the HFE or SLC17A1 genes are implicated in 95 percent of hemochromatosis patients, if you have any variants of the genes that code for such iron-overload conditions, you really have to reduce your iron intake or end up with a severe disease like hemochromatosis that can cause liver disease, joint pain, diabetes, and eye defects. So, finding out if you have these variations can be helpful. A normal person absorbs 10 percent of dietary iron; in someone with hemochromatosis, this absorption is increased threefold.

In the chart on the next page, I've listed the common sources of iron. According to the Food and Nutrition Information Center of the USDA, the recommended dietary allowance (RDA) for iron is 8 milligrams per day for males ages 19 and older, 18 milligrams per day for women between the ages of 19 to 50, and 8 milligrams per day for women ages 51 and older.[90] However, the RDA for iron in pregnant women is increased to 27 milligrams per day, as the baby in the womb will compete for the iron.

In general, for most people, a balanced, varied diet will automatically contain all the vitamins and minerals a person needs. However genomics has been both brilliant and mind-boggling in changing certain fundamental perceptions—we now know that some of us have a genetic propensity to lack or overproduce certain vitamins and minerals, and many of these traits were inherited due to the engineered nature of our evolutionary experience.

Sources of iron[91]	Amount (mg)
Heme iron (animal form)	
Chicken liver (75 g)	9.8
Lean ground chicken (75 g)	1.2
Ground beef patty (75 g)	2
Non-heme iron (plant based)	
Spinach, boiled (½ cup)	3.4
Chickpeas (¾ cup)	2.4
Tofu	1.2
Tahini (2 Tbsp)	2.7
Almonds (¼ cup)	1.5
White beans (175 ml)	5.8

Conclusion

Ultimately, the fate of our guts depends on our genes and grub—genes may not always prove fatal, but because life is a long journey, paying heed to our genomic road signs is sensible. Most of these genes are from a different era, where the fate of the human world depended on finding whatever food sources people could muster when food was scarce—and that was also a time when microbial diseases were fatal. Now we live in an era of plenty and relative safety, but with our diets becoming more and more varied, and digestive diseases worsening, it's worth understanding how to eat for our gene type without being punctilious about it.

In this book, the recurring theme has been the interaction between our genes and the environment. While our foods come from our environment, our digestive process and the ensuing metabolism creates an internal environment that our body has to deal with. In the story of Aladdin in *The Arabian Nights*, the magician had to be guided by the stars to find the boy who could exhume the lamp. Our genes are our guiding stars from our ancestral songlines, and our guts, veritable Aladdin's lamps that can brighten our daily experiences and give us immense pleasure. But every lamp needs maintenance, ensuring that the wicks or oil are clean. If we stop to think about it, our bodies are something we cannot escape from, so let's take good care of them.

Reader Rx: Food Diary

If you think you might have a food intolerance or sensitivity, it's worth it to have your genes tested to confirm. In the meantime, keep a food diary to track what foods make you feel bloated or uncomfortable. Write down everything you eat, and you will be able to find a pattern. Even for food allergies, keeping a food diary is a good method of diagnosis. Here's a sample food diary template:

Food and Drink	Quantity	Time Eaten	Symptoms/ Note

Key Points

1. Genetic variations play a big part in how people respond to different foods.
2. We know salt raises blood pressure, but this is determined by your ACE gene variant. GA or AA variants indicate high risk, whereas the GG variant does not affect your risk of developing high blood pressure due to salt intake.
3. Our ancestral origins, as hunters or pastoralists, determine our ability to digest starch; wolves cannot digest starch but dogs can.
4. Glucose is essential for cells but not essential in diets; opiate-like withdrawal symptoms occur after stopping high-sugar diets.
5. There are two ways people with a sensitivity react to gluten— a mild gluten sensitivity that causes abdominal symptoms, or a severe celiac disease where your immune system gets involved, causing a multitude of symptoms.
6. Lactose intolerance is related to the MCM6 gene, especially the CC or CT variants; if you have the TT variant, you have a low or no risk of being lactose intolerant. The origins of lactose tolerance appeared during famine in Europe when people first took to drinking cows milk in desperation; until this time, people would have found this milk toxic; during times of famine, only those that could tolerate milk survived, thereby ensuring that the milk-digesting genes traveled down the human time line.
7. Regarding vitamin A, BCMO1 is an enzyme that plays a key role in the conversion of beta-carotene into the active form of vitamin A and comes in variants AA, AG, and GG. The GG holders are poor converters and therefore need to

ensure they get enough preformed vitamin A from animal sources.

8. Iron deficiency evolved as a mechanism to protect against malaria. We know that a normal person absorbs 10 percent of dietary iron; in someone with the genetic tendency for hemochromatosis, this absorption is increased threefold.

9. The fate of our bodies depends on our genes, diets, and environment—genes may not always prove fatal, but eating according to our gene type can help boost our wellness.

CONCLUSION

EAT, MOVE, LIVE

The root of all health is in the brain.
The trunk of it is in emotion.
The branches and leaves are the body.
The flower of health blooms
when all parts work together.

—Kurdish saying

In some ways this book is a curated exposition of living well—a retrospective of guts, genes, and geography and their impact on good health—a brief history of human evolution, genetic restlessness, and the power of positive thought.

Western medicine has weapons that can torpedo tumors and vaccinate against viruses. Eastern medicine works on the energy of faith, using consciousness to bring wholesomeness to our individual bodily constitutions. Many years ago, I trekked in the Himalayas. My second novel, *To Kill a Snow Dragonfly*, was set in Tibet. The Tibetans have a concept of rLung—"wind" or "breath," that has a remarkable philosophical equivalence to the Greek *pneuma*, Chinese *qi*, or Ayurvedic *prana*—life forces or vital energies that bind all life-forms. Tibetans use an elegant image of a tree to illustrate health—the tree of health has only two kinds of fruit and flowers, indicating good outcomes: the two flowers are said to be freedom from disease and increased longevity, and the fruits are spiritual and material well-being. In other words, without good health, there can be no happiness or enjoyment of material things.

Western medicine has a certain clinical detachment, a feeling that any application of science requires an absence of sentiment. Touching is strictly for examination. In Eastern medicine, touching is not necessarily a trespassing of boundaries but a natural human construct.

After all, touch is the only sense essential for being. The other senses—vision, hearing, taste, and smell—exist for well-being but are not essential for survival. Touch is indispensable for all life-forms. Even bacteria exhibit contact inhibition, a form of touch. A study done on the C. elegans worms showed that physical interaction with other worms improved growth and development.

In 1986, Tiffany Field and colleagues studied twenty preterm babies—one group received fifteen minutes of touch three times a day; the other group was not touched, in keeping with prevailing views about causing infections.[1] The study showed that the touched group gained twice as much weight and were able to be discharged from the hospital earlier.

Decades ago, the psychologist Sidney Jourard had studied the importance of touch and advocated touch therapy. While his work gained popularity after his death, and touch and energy healing became widespread, touch and touch therapy do not stack up in double-blind controlled clinical trials. In fact, the youngest person to publish a paper in the prestigious *JAMA*, the eleven-year-old Emily Rosa, studied over two hundred energy healers and found more than half could not detect the presence or absence of a nearby body. In her study, healers put hands through a curtain and recorded when they felt Emily's hand alongside theirs.[2] This led to touch therapy being ridiculed by mainstream medicine. But do nondrug or nonsurgical interventions need to pass such rigorous scrutiny? Or is it a matter of faith? After all, a significant proportion of humanity believes in an unseen creator; where there is faith, there is hope. Faith matters. Humanity needs hope. Ultimately it isn't about East or West, but our own individual responsibility, a sense of purpose about our own lives. Just as law isn't always about justice, medicine isn't always about health. Hope and faith are seeds that can give rise to change.

Ted Kaptchuk of Harvard Medical School continues to study the power of faith in clinical studies. I mentioned Ted's migraine and acupuncture studies earlier. Pain is a good warning system, and placebos are useful as evolutionary mirrors held up to treat phantom pain.

We now know that placebo drugs cannot shrink tumors or eliminate viruses, but they can stimulate real physiological responses, from changes in heart rate and blood pressure to chemical activity in the brain, helping pain, depression, anxiety, fatigue, and even some symptoms of Parkinson's. That's why the power of the mind matters and the stress response is stupendous. Stress cannot cause a tumor, but it can make the outcome worse after you develop one, as I've seen in my patients. Stress is a powerful drug that we can use, if we learn to avoid it lingering for too long.

That's why, as we noted in the chapters on stress and anxiety, these stress genes that endured evolutionary time actually ensured the survival of our species. So what's wrong with harnessing our own finely honed psychological powers of persuasion toward physical or physiological ends? Faith, hope, and loving touch can translate to perceptual, authentic, and existential living.

When Darwin noted different skin colors in different continents, he didn't realize the impact of our diets. Unlike animals, humans changed their diets due to climate, circumstance, and continental migration. After diets were accounted for, Inuit skin darkened over time and Baltic bodies lightened due to the need for vitamin D. We know that saturated fat intake makes very little difference to cholesterol levels, provided diets are constant and made up of varied food types. Processed foods, with their high trans fats, and fructose sugar have practically spawned a new species. But expecting medicine or surgery to solve the weight problems so many now deal with is both unrealistic and untenable. We cannot ingest unhealthy foods and expect wellness in return.

Food is food. There is no need for guilt around what we eat; we simply need to understand what we eat becomes us eventually. We are what we eat. We've covered fat guts and skinny brains. We are bright enough to see we are damaging the planet but not sensible enough to change it. Clearly, we feel that we are the top of the evolutionary pyramid, but even nature's wish to see each creature grow and thrive can be thwarted by progress that excludes our environment in our decision-making process. Ultimately, every species in the world is dispensable. Look at the evidence: dinosaurs, saber-toothed cats, wooly mammoths.

Aha, you think. *To eat well, and to be true to our bodies, we have to be logical with some scientific scheming. No diets for me, folks. Yes, sir. I don't care about dieting competitions or nips and tucks. It's all to do with my brain.* But evolution is crafty by nature. "Hold on," it says, "let me check your genome to see which gene applies to you." It's rather like checking a biological penal code to see which scientific statute applies to you or which crime you are guilty of. This is because nature has allowed itself the indulgence of making individuals within each species, by surreptitiously encoding our dietary destiny within our genes.

Genes are neither compassionate nor cruel, but simply end up in the bodies of certain creatures they won't mind eliminating. Just as genes shape the environment, the environment shapes our genes. Human beings have overpopulated all corners of the planet and plundered resources simply thinking that if we stop doing things to damage the environment, nature will go back to the way it was—

waters would freeze again, reefs will rebuild, and extinct species can become extant again. Whether we like it or not, a future is coming where the natural will no longer be natural, and with replaceable parts humans may indeed no longer be fully human, so we can ill afford to forget our roots. There is a saying in India that even a lotus flower is stuck in mud. We cannot escape evolutionary quicksand. To survive, we have to keep moving, thinking, giving, and eating sensibly, thereby allowing our genes to express freely.

Big data, genomics, biometrics—the future is here. Soon we'll be personalizing our healthcare to suit individual needs. It will be a world where man shall attempt to rebel against the domination of evolution. In our cities, we may have technology, but we cannot be masters of the intricate machinery that exists inside our cells. In their communications with each other, our cells have established great communication channels and the ability to cope with nature. There may be a message here for humanity itself.

In each of the chapters on stress, sluggishness, and obesity, we can see the overlapping messages: movement is good; generosity helps; stress is bad; sugar, especially fructose, is filthy. Moderation is good when we want to put something inside our bodies, as our cells and genes then need to digest or detoxify what we ingest. Exuberance is good when we want to live. In my medical career, I've dealt with a lot of skin cancer—melanomas afflict young and old. I've never met someone who, at the end of life, regretted not buying another car or failing to marry another spouse. From these conversations I've learned that life is ultimately about what we give, not what we take, and what we make, not what we break (including relationships). Life is a biological creation, so let's embrace the unbiased beauty of science and enjoy living to the fullest.

Soon, prescribing drugs according to our gene types will become the norm. That in itself is a method of tackling illness in ways we have never tried before. It's like being an athlete and preparing for the Olympic games. I went to observe elite athletes undergoing specialized and personalized training before the recent Rio Olympics. In events such as the Olympics, with its great history, merely training hard isn't enough to succeed. Historical performance and personal bests are tendentious at best. What you need is a history of what has worked and what hasn't worked for you and others; next, you need to know your body and metabolic function. Then, a training program or specialized equipment needs can be created for your body measurements. This is what leads to better performance and success in the future. That's what *The Genetics of Health* is ultimately all about.

Scientists have now mapped the entire human DNA and even developed techniques to modify or edit genes. To me, gene expression by our own actions and diets is natural; gene editing isn't. The former requires thought and action; the latter has a certain level of detachment from the evolutionary scheme of things that may prove unwise. We are now painting the future of mankind—with brushes of faith and pigments of our scientific imaginations. Evolution is a self-programming system that molds the finest creations. Gene editing—replacing defective genes—is merely making humans lab rats that can only exist in a two-dimensional realm: feeding and being fed. True science not only has an inquiring mind, but it also understands our place in the universe. That's what this journey has taught me.

On my own long walkabout, I watched the evolutionary train chugging along, the stress response serving as its shadowy conductor—confident, precise, and making sure to communicate with all passengers. The trains were automated and punctual. None of the passengers have any control over their journey or destination. The food on board the train is sweet, plentiful, processed, and delicious. Everyone has an allocated seat and walking around is almost impossible due to overcrowding. People seem sincere, but they also seem to have no choice but to obey their financial masters. There is a general feeling of disenfranchisement.

While I practice evidence-based medicine, I'm never one to dismiss alternative or complementary therapies that patients want to try. Just because you don't really get it or the science doesn't stack up, it does not mean you have to be dismissive. If people or patients don't feel acknowledged, then you can't feel authentic to them or be a guide or teacher. After all, the word *doctor* derives from *docere* in Latin: to teach. Saint Augustine said, "Faith is to believe what you do not see; the reward of this faith is to see what you believe."[3] We must acknowledge the power of our minds and know its power. Everything is possible if we believe and hope. That's why it's never too late to be positive or become healthy. Nelson Mandela spent twenty-seven years in prison, many of them in solitary confinement. He was in prison for almost as long as I've been a doctor. Yet in his autobiography, Mandela wrote: "I am fundamentally an optimist. Whether that comes from nature or nurture, I cannot say. Part of being optimistic is keeping one's head pointed toward the sun, one's feet moving forward."[4] That's sensible advice for health and living life.

Last year, I was awarded the Ko Awatea International Excellence Award for Leading Health Improvement on a Global Scale. It was at the Asia Pacific Forum (APAC), the largest medical gathering in this region. I felt it deeply humbling when the citation said it was for practicing "patient-centered medicine" on a global scale, as most of my work has been in lower socioeconomic communities and any "leadership" on my part has been purely accidental. At the awards ceremony, many people in the media and my medical colleagues asked me about my daily regimen, diet, and mechanisms to deal with stress. Everyone thinks I'm impossibly busy, look younger than my age, and always seem positive. I'm not sure I have any magic formula, but I reckon these four things help: working, learning, moving, and giving.

François Rabelais wrote, "Without health life is not life, it is not living life. Without health life is only a languishment and an image of death."[5] I've often said all people can be classified into three types based on their beliefs: Judeo-Christian and Islamic, with beliefs in heaven or hell; Eastern, Hindus and Buddhists, with beliefs in reincarnation; or greenie atheists who get recycled by earthworms with no afterlife. But every *body* gets only one go. In this life on earth we are given, what we do in this life really matters. So let's make our actions count.

The way I see it, birth and death are merely doors that open into the grand hall of life—a life furnished with comfy memories, draped with love of family and friends, and carpets worn by the footfalls of our many travels. Our lives may be our grand ballrooms, but our bodies are the rooms we cannot escape from and they need looking after.

Our bodies are essentially carriers of genes, which is why most cancers and diseases like dementia occur after our reproductive peaks have been passed. Genes may be our blueprints, and in the proteins they express exists our responsibility toward the future—for us and others. If we share two-thirds of our genes with a lowly worm, nature has given us some genetic wiggle room. With our actions and diets, as I've stressed in this book, we can make real changes in our gene expression. Genes are like miniature master chefs, valuing simplicity but giving diners plenty of options. Our genetic ingredients are not sacred; what we can create using them is. Life is ultimately a tasting platter—one that we must depart nourished rather than uncomfortably full.

This book is about the science of health, i.e., living well. Medicine is a complex narrative of human industry and scientific zeal, in a world full of disease, real and imagined. When genes were mapped, everyone assumed humanity would be reduced to binary code, we'd become digital humans living our imaginary lives. But these small and selfish groupies, genes, end up as microscopic mapmakers of our history. We have to embrace humanity's backstory and heredity, even if we cannot change it. Evolution may be complicated and messy, but we cannot turn our backs on it. Good health needs some creative work—a sense of aerobicized deter-mination combined with knowledge of our genetic history, while allowing heredity the respect to shape our health and happiness

---

Reader Rx: Testing Your Genes

Towards understanding our blueprints better, I've developed the R$_x$evolution 21-Gene Testing Program® that can analyze your genetic code (from saliva samples) and determine how your genes can influence your stress levels, nutrient or mineral metabolism, and sports preferences. Most importantly, as discussed in this book, you can learn to eat for your gene type. If you wish to order this test, and receive a personalized report, further details are on this book's website: www.genet icsofhealth.com.

ACKNOWLEDGMENTS

For a writer, the act of putting pen to paper is a conversation—"we talk to ourselves, we do." What the reader ultimately reads is not imagination but simulation because, for a writer, nothing is sacred—friends, family, and clients find their way onto pages in sometimes unrecognizable forms. If writers weren't allowed to use any human within their orbit as material, a writer would be forced to live in solitary confinement. Therefore, writers make unspoken but impassioned requests of their friends and family. After all, one must still go through hours and hours of rewrites, edits, anger, and rejections before one gets the privilege of getting published. They did not ask questions about my late nights hunched in front of a keyboard, typing with two fingers.

We now live in an era where Dr. Google has become the world's most famous diagnostician of diseases. Medicine used to cause interesting epistemological mayhem and epidemiological madness before the internet. Now we don't diagnose diseases—our brains merely download them from data we collate. If we think of medicine as a specialized pursuit, it has come at a price. Doctors are no longer philosophers and thinkers, and sometimes they're not even scientists.

There are a few people I must thank; there are many others I should but don't have room on these pages, so a sheepish and collective thank-you to everyone who has supported me over the years.

To my parents, Samadhanam and Lily—I owe you everything, especially gratitude for teaching me that the most important part of medicine is being human; to my loving daughter, Natasha, for allowing me to pretend to be grown up and enlightened; to Sunita, for making stories of geriatric patients sound radically compelling; to my staff nurses, Wendy and Lanzy, for managing my practice so wonderfully well; to the "walking group"—you know who you are; to my patients, for helping me learn daily lessons and thereby become better; to my editorial team at Beyond Words—for sacrificing a few of my darlings in the spirit of this writing adventure; to the Merrin family, especially Mom Lee; to Bill G., my agent in America and Barbara T., publicist— thank you all, from the bottom of my heart. And finally, to Zack, for reminding me about the canine capacity for unconditional love. I do forgive you for eating bits of this manuscript.

NOTES

INTRODUCTION

1. David Wroth, "Star-Dreaming—Seven Sisters," *Aboriginal Art Stories*, Japingka Gallery, accessed June 1, 2016, http://www.japingka.com.au/articles/star-dreaming-seven-sisters.
2. Bryan Sykes, *The Seven Daughters of Eve: The Science that Reveals Our Genetic Ancestry* (London: Corgi Books, 2002), 336–338.
3. James Vance Marshall, *Walkabout* (London: Puffin, 1979), 57.
4. Oprah Winfrey, AZ Quotes, accessed August 25, 2016, http://www.azquotes.com/quote/318161.

CHAPTER 1

1. Juha Huhtakangas et al., "Effect of Increased Warfarin Use on Warfarin-Related Cerebral Hemorrhage: A Longitudinal Population-Based Study," *Stroke* 42, no. 9 (September 2011): 2431–2435. http://stroke.ahajournals.org/content/42/9/2431.
2. Richard Dawkins, *The Selfish Gene* (Oxford: Oxford University Press, 1989), 33.
3. Richard Dawkins, *The Extended Phenotype: The Gene as the Unit of Selection* (Oxford: Oxford University Press, 1989), xiii.
4. Richard Dawkins, *The Selfish Gene* (Oxford: Oxford University Press, 1989), 3.
5. Jenny Santi, "The Science Behind the Power of Giving," *Live Science* (December 1, 2015) http://www.livescience.com/52936-need-to-give-boosted-by-brain-science-and-evolution.html.
6. Charles Darwin, *The Descent of Man and Selection in Relation to Sex*, 2nd ed. (London, 1874), 98.

7. Daniel Stimson, "Inner Workings of the Magnanimous Mind," *National Institutes of Neurological Disorders and Stroke*, April 4, 2007: http://www.ninds.nih.gov/news_and_events/news_articles/brain_activity_during_altruism.htm.

8. Hilary Davidson and Christian Smith, *The Paradox of Generosity: Giving We Receive, Grasping We Lose* (Oxford: Oxford University Press, 2014).

9. Peter Kokkinos, *Physical Activity and Cardiovascular Disease Prevention* (Boston: Jones & Bartlett Learning, 2010), 311.

10. Public Library of Science, "α +-Thalassemia and Protection from Malaria," *PLoS Medicine* 3, no. 5 (May 2006): e221. http://www.ncbi.nlm.nih.gov/pmc/articles/PMC1435782/.

11. Dean Ornish, "Changing Lifestyle Changes Gene Expression: A Talk with Dean Ornish," Edge, December 3, 2008: https://www.edge.org/conversation/dean_ornish-changing-lifestyle-changes-gene-expression.

12. David Derbyshire, "Why Acupuncture Is Giving Skeptics the Needle," *The Guardian*, July 26, 2013, https://www.theguardian.com/science/2013/jul/26/acupuncture-sceptics-proof-effective-nhs.

13. Ibid.

14. Charlotte Paterson et al., "Acupuncture for 'Frequent Attenders' with Medically Unexplained Symptoms," *The British Journal of General Practice* 61, no. 587 (June 2011): 295–305. https://www.ncbi.nlm.nih.gov/pmc/articles/PMC3103692.

15. Tia Ghose, "Placebo's Effect May Depend on Your Genes," LiveScience.com, October 23, 2012, http://www.livescience.com/24222-placebo-effect-genes.html.

16. For further reading on this subject, researchers Regmi and Bharati from Nepal have an excellent summary of genetic variations and the drugs they affect: Laxman Bharati and Balmukunda Regmi, "Genetic Variation in Drug Disposition," in *Readings in Advanced Pharmacokinetics—Theory, Methods and Applications*, ed. Dr. Ayman Noreddin (Rijeka, Croatia: InTech, 2012): 101–110.

CHAPTER 2

1. M. Rottensteiner et al., "Physical Activity, Fitness, Glucose Homeostasis, and Brain Morphology in Twins," *Medicine and Science in Sports and Exercise* 47, no. 3 (March 2015): 509–518.

2. Kevin Loria, "Scientists Discovered What Happens When One Twin Exercises and the Other Does Not," *Business Insider*, March 11, 2015, http://www.businessinsider.com/twin-study-shows-exercise-effects-on-brain-and-body-2015-3.

3. Rachel Brown, "Couch Potato Gene Found in Mice, Says Study," *BioNews* 743 (February 24, 2014): http://www.bionews.org.uk/page_399230.asp.

4. Fred H. Previc, *The Dopaminergic Mind in Human Evolution and History* (Cambridge: Cambridge University Press, 2011).

5. Emiliana Borrelli et al., "Epigenetic Reprogramming of Cortical Neurons through Alteration of Dopaminergic Circuits," *Molecular Psychiatry* 19, no. 11 (2014): 1193–1200.

6. Haruki Murakami, *1Q84: A Novel* (New York: Knopf, 2009): 29.

7. Sharad Paul, "The Myth of Race," TEDx Auckland, *YouTube* (July 6, 2016): 18:10. https://www.youtube.com/watch?v=d6ru05esR1U.

8. Daniel Wolpert, "The Real Reason for Brains," TEDGlobal (July 2011): 19:59. https://www.ted.com/talks/daniel_wolpert_the_real_reason_for_brains?language=en.

9. Dennis M. Bramble and Daniel E. Lieberman, "Endurance Running and the Evolution of *Homo*," *Nature* 432, no. 7015 (2004): 345–352.

10. David A. Raichlen and J. D. Polk, "Linking Brains and Brawn: Exercise and the Evolution of Human Neurobiology," *Proceedings of the Royal Society of London B: Biological Sciences* 280, no. 1750 (2013): doi: 10.1098/rspb.2012.2250.

11. Vera Nazarian, *The Perpetual Calendar of Inspiration: Old Wisdom for a New World* (Highgate, VT: Spirit, 2010), April 10.

12. Alexander G. Liu, "Haootia quadriformis n. gen., n. sp., Interpreted as Muscular Cnidarian Impression from the Late Ediacaran Period (approx. 560 Ma)," *Proceedings of the Royal Society B* (August 27, 2014): doi: 10.1098/rspb.2014.1202.

13. Evan Eichler et al., "Evolution of Human-Specific Neural SRGAP2 Genes by Incomplete Segmental Duplication," *Cell* 149, no. 4 (2012): 912–922.

14. David Carrier, "The Advantage of Standing Up to Fight and the Evolution of Habitual Bipedalism in Hominins," *PLoS ONE* 6 (May 18, 2014): e19630.

15. Sir Francis Bacon, "L. Of Studies," in *The Works of Francis Bacon, Lord Chancellor of England*, ed. Basil Montagu (Philadelphia: Carey and Hart, 1848), 55.

16. Mark Twain, *The Quote Garden*, accessed Aug 21, 2016, www.quotegarden.com/exercise.html.

17. J. B. S. Haldane, "On Being the Right Size," in *Possible Worlds: And Other Essays* (London: Chatto and Windus, 1927), 19.

18. Confucius, in *Short Sayings of Great Men*, ed. Samuel Arthur Bent (Boston: Ticknor and Company, 1882), 159.

19. Gregory Steinberg, in "From Athlete to Couch Potato: What 2 Missing Genes May Mean," Jennifer Welsh, *LiveScience*, September 5, 2011, http://www.livescience.com/15905-lazy-active-genes.html.

20. Katarzyna Bozek and Yuning Wei et al., "Exceptional Evolutionary Divergence of Human Muscle and Brain Metabolomes Parallels Human Cognitive and Physical Uniqueness," *PLoS Biol* 12, no. 5 (May 27, 2014): e1001871.

21. Ibid., e1001871. doi:10.1371/journal.pbio.1001871.

22. Friedrich Nietzsche, *Nietzsche: Imagery and Thought: A Collection of Essays*, ed. Malcolm Pasley (Oakland, California: University of California Press, 1978), 118.

23. Isabell Petrinic, "Study's Findings Are Music to the Ears of Dancers," *The Daily Telegraph*, March 23, 2016, http://www.dailytelegraph.com.au/newslocal/west/studys-findings-are-music-to-the-ears-of-dancers/news-story/213c5423e5fc78eaf1da04b466581a42.

24. G. R. Nalcakan, "The Effects of Sprint Interval vs. Continuous Endurance Training on Physiological and Metabolic Adaptations in Young Healthy Adults," *Journal of Human Kinetics* 44 (2014): 97–109: https://www.ncbi.nlm.nih.gov/pmc/articles/PMC4327385/.

25. Dan Buettner, "The Island Where People Forget to Die," *The New York Times Magazine*, October 24, 2012, http://www.nytimes.com/2012/10/28/magazine/the-island-where-people-forget-to-die.html?_r=0.

26. Dan Buettner, *The Blue Zones Solution: Eating and Living Like the World's Healthiest People* (New York: National Geographic Books, 2015).

27. D. Craig Willcox et al., "Genetic Determinants of Exceptional Human Longevity: Insights from the Okinawa Centenarian Study," *Age* 20, no. 4 (December 2006): 313–332. https://www.ncbi.nlm.nih.gov/pmc/articles/PMC3259160/.

28. Richard P. Ebstein et al., "*AVPR1a* and *SLC6A4* Gene Polymorphisms Are Associated with Creative Dance Performance," *Public Library of Science Genetics* 1, no. 3 (2005): e42.

29. Joe Verghese et al., "Leisure Activities and the Risk of Dementia in the Elderly," *New England Journal of Medicine* 348 (2003): 2508–2516.

30. University of Strathclyde and Caledonian University, "Medical Proof of SCD Being Good for Health," *RSCDS Members' Magazine* (October 2010): 12, http://web.rscds-falkirk.org.uk/about/health/Proof_SCD_is_Good_for_You.html.

31. Oliver Sacks, *Awakenings* (New York: Vintage, 1999): 9.

32. Madeleine Hackney et al., "Health-Related Quality of Life and Alternative Forms of Exercise in Parkinson Disease," *Parkinsonism & Related Disorders* 15, no. 9 (2009): 644–648.

33. Amy Packham, "Fascinating 4D Scan Video Shows Babies Reacting to Music in Womb in 'First Study' of Its Kind," *The Huffington Post*, August 10, 2015, http://www.huffingtonpost.co.uk/2015/10/08/babies-reacting-music-in-womb-singing-_n_8261782.html.

34. Gammon M. Earhart, "Dance as Therapy for Individuals with Parkinson Disease," *European Journal of Physical and Rehabilitation Medicine* 45, no. 2 (2009): 231–238.

35. Carol V. Ward, "Interpreting the Posture and Locomotion of Australopithecus afarensis: Where Do We Stand?" *American Journal of Physical Anthropology* 19, no. 35 (2002): 195–215.

36. Lawrence M. Parsons, "The Neural Basis of Human Dance," *Cerebral Cortex* 16, no. 8 (2006): 1157–1167.

37. Patrick Q. Page, "Phantom at the Opera," *Early Edition*, season 1, episode 20, directed by Jan Eliasberg, aired April 19, 1997 (Los Angeles: CBS, 1997).

38. Terry Pratchett, "Sir Terry Pratchett—Dementia Blog, What's the Point of It All?" *Alzheimer's Research UK Blog*, September 17, 2013, http://www.dementiablog.org/terry-pratchett-on-dementia/.

39. Mei Chen et al., "Cadherin-11 Regulates Fibroblast Inflammation," *Proceedings of the National Academy of Sciences* 108, no. 20 (2011): 8402–8407.

40. Koichi Ando et al., "Analysis of N-cadherin Interacting Proteins in Alzheimer's Disease," *Alzheimer's & Dementia* 6, no. 4 (2010): S403.

41. Ian Sample, "Neanderthals Were Not Less Intelligent than Modern Humans, Scientists Find," *The Guardian*, April 30, 2014, https://www.theguardian.com/science/2014/apr/30/neanderthals-not-less-intelligent-humans-scientists.

42. Calvin Newport, "The Procrastinating Caveman: What Human Evolution Teaches Us about Why We Put Off Work and How to Stop," *Cal Newport*, July 10, 2011, http://calnewport.com/blog/2011/07/10/the-procrastinating-caveman-what-human -evolution-teaches-us-about-why-we-put-off-work-and-how-to-stop/.

43. Ibid.

44. Ibid.

45. Yan Wu, "Individual Differences in Resting-State Functional Connectivity Predict Procrastination," *Personality and Individual Differences* 95 (2016): 62–67.

46. Cedric Ginestet, "The Unbearable Lightness of Procrastination," *Psychologist* 18, no. 8 (2005): 480.

47. Daniel Gustavson et al., "Genetic Relations among Procrastination, Impulsivity, and Goal-Management Ability: Implications for the Evolutionary Origin of Procrastination," *Psychological Science* 25, no. 6 (2014): 1178–1188.

48. Piers Steel, *The Procrastination Equation: How to Stop Putting Things Off and Start Getting Stuff Done* (New York: Harper Perennial, 2012): 52.

49. Sir Francis Galton, *Inquiries into Human Faculty and Its Development* (London: Macmillan & Co., 1883): 155–173.

50. Association for Psychological Science, "Procrastination and Impulsivity Genetically Linked: Exploring the Genetics of 'I'll do It Tomorrow,'" *ScienceDaily* website, April 7 2014, www.sciencedaily.com/releases/2014/04/140407101718.htm.

51. Rodolphe Töpffer, *Enter the Comics: Rodolphe Töpffer's Essay on Physiognomy and The True Story of Monsieur Crépin*, ed. Ellen Wiese (Lincoln: University of Nebraska Press, 1965).

CHAPTER 3

1. George Bernard Shaw, Quotes.net, accessed August 21, 2016, http://www.quotes.net/ quote/420.

2. Elizabeth Kostova, *The Historian* (New York: Little, Brown and Company, 2005), ix.

3. Melissa Hogenboom, "The Lucy Fossil Rewrote the Story of Humanity," *Earth by BBC* (November 27, 2014), http://www.bbc.com/earth/story/20141127-lucy-fossil -revealed-our-origins.

4. William Blake, "The Tyger," *Songs of Innocence and of Experience, Copy Z* (London: William Blake, 1826): 42.

5. R. M. Nesse and G. C. Williams, *Why We Get Sick: The New Science of Darwinian Medicine* (New York: Vintage, 1994).

6. Charles Darwin, "Instinct," *The Origin of Species* (London: John Murray, 1859): 244.

7. Randolph Nesse, in *Useful Fictions: Evolution, Anxiety and the Origins of Literature*, Michael Austin (Lincoln: University of Nebraska Press, 2010).

8. Robert-Paul Juster and Marie-France Marin, "Genetics and Stress: Is There a Link?" *Mammoth Magazine* 9 (January 2011): 1–2, http://www.humanstress.ca/documents/ pdf/Mammouth%20Magazine/Mammoth_vol9_EN.pdf.

9. Michael Meaney et al., "Environmental Programming of Stress Responses through DNA Methylation: Life at the Interface between a Dynamic Environment and a Fixed Genome," *Dialogues in Clinical Neuroscience* 7, no. 2 (2005): 103–23.

10. K. S. Kendler et al., "Childhood Parental Loss and Adult Psychopathology in Women. A Twin Study Perspective," *Archives of General Psychiatry* 49, no. 2 (1992): 109–116.

11. Joohyung Lee et al., "The Male Fight-Flight Response: A Result of SRY Regulation of Catecholamines?" *Bioessays* 34, no. 6 (2012): 454–457.

12. Robert-Paul Juster and Marie-France Marin, "Genetics and Stress: Is There a Link?" *Mammoth Magazine* 9 (January 2011): 1–2.

13. Nassim Nicholas Taleb, "Stretch of the Imagination," *New Statesman*, December 2, 2010, http://www.newstatesman.com/ideas/2010/11/box-procrustes-call-bed-taleb.

14. Daniel Defoe, *Robinson Crusoe* (Oxford: Oxford University Press, 2007), 130.

15. David Kohn, *The Darwinian Heritage* (Princeton, NJ: Princeton University Press, 2014), 588.

16. Ralph Colp Jr, *To Be an Invalid: The Illness of Charles Darwin* (Chicago: University of Chicago, 1977), 228.

17. Stephen King, *On Writing: A Memoir of the Craft* (New York: Scribner, 2010), 29.

18. Ibid, 150.

19. T. J. Barloon et al., "Charles Darwin and Panic Disorder," *Journal of the American Medical Association* 277, no. 2 (1997): 138–41.

20. Walter B. Cannon, *The Wisdom of the Body* (New York: W. W. Norton & Company, Inc., 1932).

21. Cassandra Clare, *City of Lost Souls* (New York: Margaret K. McElderry Books, 2012), 423.

22. Martin Maripuu et al., "Relative Hypo- and Hypercortisolism Are Both Associated with Depression and Lower Quality of Life in Bipolar Disorder: A Cross-Sectional Study," *PLoS ONE* 9, no. 6 (2014): e98682.

23. Dieferson da Costa Estrela et al., "Predictive Behaviors for Anxiety and Depression in Female Wistar Rats Subjected to Cafeteria Diet and Stress," *Physiology & Behavior* 151 (2015): 252–263.

24. Harriet Grove, *Anne Grey: A Novel*, ed. T. H. Lister (Paris: Baudry's European Library, 1834), 48.

25. Spyridon Koulouris et al., "Takotsubo Cardiomyopathy: The 'Broken Heart' Syndrome," *Hellenic Journal of Cardiology* 51 (2010): 451–457.

26. Janet Torpy et al., "Chronic Stress and the Heart," *Journal of the American Medical Association* 298, no. 14 (2007): 1722.

27. Charles Dickens, *Barnaby Rudge* (London: Wordsworth Editions Limited, 1998), 174.

28. P. Schuck, "Glycated Hemoglobin as a Physiological Measure of Stress and Its Relation to Some Psychological Stress Indicators," *Behavioral Medicine* 24, no. 2 (1998): 89–94.

29. George Orwell, *The Collected Essays, Journalism and Letters of George Orwell: In Front of Your Nose, 1945–1950*, vol. 4, eds. Sonia Orwell and Ian Angus (New York: Harcourt, Brace & World, 1968), 515.

30. Joachim Fuchsberger. *Altwerden ist nichts für Feiglinge* (Germany: Gütersloher Verlagshaus, 2011).

31. Anne Marie Lykkegaard, "Metabolism Works Differently Than We Thought," *Science Nordic*, March 18, 2014, http://sciencenordic.com/metabolism-works-differently -we-thought.

32. Antoine Lavoisier, "Alterations qu'éprouve l'air respiré: Recueil des memoires de Lavoisier," (1785), read to the Societé de Médicine and reprinted as part of *Mémoires sur la respiration et la transpiration des animaux in Les maîtres de la pensée scientifique* (Paris: Gauthier-Villaus, 1920).

33. Howard Murad, *Conquering Cultural Stress: The Ultimate Guide to Anti-Aging and Happiness* (Los Angeles: Wisdom Waters Press, 2015), 16.

34. Kristian Sjøgren, "Your Face Reveals Risk of Heart Attack," ScienceNordic.com, December 6, 2012, http://sciencenordic.com/your-face-reveals-risk-heart-attack.

35. W. T. Blows, "Neurotransmitters of the Brain: Serotonin, Noradrenaline (Norepinephrine), and Dopamine," *Journal of Neuroscience Nursing* 32, no. 4 (2000): 234–238.

36. M. Hajos et al., "Reduced Responsiveness of Locus Coeruleus Neurons to Cutaneous Thermal Stimuli in Capsaicin-Treated Rats," *Neuroscience Letters* 70, no. 3 (1986): 382–387.

37. Jean Francois Fernel, *De Naturali Parte Medicinae Libri Septem* (France, 1542), 1.

38. Anthony Kenny, *Descartes: A Study of His Philosophy* (New York: Random House, 1968), 64.

39. C. L. Moraes et al., "Interplay between Glutamate and Serotonin within the Dorsal Periaqueductal Gray Modulates Anxiety-Related Behavior of Rats Exposed to the Elevated Plus-Maze," *Behavioral Brain Research* 194, no. 2 (2008): 181–186.

40. Umami Information Center, "Report on the Umami Symposium at the European Sensory Network Seminar in Porto, Portugal, 9 May 2007," accessed March 1, 2016, http://www.umamiinfo.com/2007/06/the-appliance-of-science-1.php.

41. Alexandra Sifferlin, "Is the Link between Depression and Serotonin a Myth?" *TIME Magazine*, April 21, 2015, http://time.com/3829565/is-the-link-between -depression-and-serotonin-a-myth/.

42. Jonathan Leo and Jeffrey Lacasse, "Serotonin and Depression: A Disconnect between the Advertisements and the Scientific Literature," *PLoS Medicine* 2, no. 12 (2005): e392.

43. Susannah E. Murphy et al., "Tryptophan Supplementation Induces a Positive Bias in the Processing of Emotional Material in Healthy Female Volunteers," *Psychopharmacology* 187, no. 1 (2006): 121–130.

44. B. H. Lerner, "Can Stress Cause Disease? Revisiting the Tuberculosis Research of Thomas Holmes, 1949-1961," *Annals of Internal Medicine* 124, no. 7 (April 1, 1996): 673–80.

45. Suzanne C. Segerstrom and G. E. Miller, "Psychological Stress and the Human Immune System: A Meta-Analytic Study of 30 Years of Inquiry," *Psychological Bulletin* 130, no. 4 (2004): 601–630.

46. World Health Organization, *Global Tuberculosis Report* (Geneva: World Health Organization, 2012): 1. http://www.who.int/tb/publications/global_report/gtbr12_main.pdf.

47. Ronald Glaser et al., "Stress-Induced Immunomodulation: Implications for Tumorigenesis," *Brain, Behavior, and Immunity* 17, no. 1 (2003): 37–40.

48. "Glaser, M. Ronald PhD," *The Ohio State University: Cancer Biology and Genetics,* http://medicine.osu.edu/mvimg/directory/molecular-virology/glaser-m-ronald-phd /Pages/index.aspx.

49. Arthur C. Clarke, "Nine Billion Names of God," in *Star Science Fiction Stories No. 1 Anthology,* ed. Frederick Pohl (New York: Ballantine Books, 1953), 1.

50. John Hoey, "Of Genes and Stars," *Canadian Medical Association Journal* 163, no. 4 (2000): 381.

51. John Green, *The Fault in Our Stars* (New York: Penguin, 2013), 20.

52. Charles Letourneau, *Physiologie des Passions* (Paris: C. Reinwald & Cie, 1878), 79.

53. Thierry Steimer, "The Biology of Fear- and Anxiety-Related Behaviors," *Dialogues in Clinical Neuroscience* 4, no. 3 (2002): 231–249.

54. Steve Ramirez et al., "Activating Positive Memory Engrams Suppresses Depression-Like Behaviour," *Nature* 522, no. 7556 (2015): 335–339.

55. Martin E. P. Seligman, *Learned Optimism: How to Change Your Mind and Your Life* (New York: Vintage, 2011), 211.

56. Peter Schulman, "Applying Learned Optimism to Increase Sales Productivity," *Journal of Personal Selling & Sales Management* xix, no. 1 (winter 1999): 31–37.

57. Suzanne C. Segerstrom, "Optimism and Immunity: Do Positive Thoughts Always Lead to Positive Effects?" *Brain, Behavior, and Immunity* 19, no. 3 (2005): 195–200.

58. Deepak Chopra, *The Book of Secrets: Unlocking the Hidden Dimensions of Your Life* (New York: Harmony, 2005), 97.

59. Dalai Lama, in "11 Quotes from the Dalai Lama That'll Make You a Better Person," Wordables.com, accessed August 25, 2016, http://wordables.com/quotes-from-the -dalai-lama/.

60. Ivan Pavlov, *Oeuvres Choisies* (Moscow: Moscou, 1954), 250–251.

61. Aniko Korosi and T. Z. Baram, "The Pathways from Mother's Love to Baby's Future," *Frontiers in Behavioral Neuroscience* 3, no 27 (2009): pages 1–8.

62. Aparna Suvrathan et al., "Stress Enhances Fear by Forming New Synapses with Greater Capacity for Long-Term Potentiation in the Amygdala," *Philosophical Transactions of the Royal Society B: Biological Sciences* 369 (2013): 1633.

63. Shannon Harvey, "How to Change Your Brain's Stress Response," *The Connection,* February 19, 2015, https://theconnection.tv/change-brains-stress-response/.

64. Contzen Pereira, "Music Enhances Cognitive-Related Behaviour in Snails," *Journal of Entomology and Zoology Studies* 3, no. 5 (2015): 379–386.

65. Wendy Koreyva, "Learn to Meditate in 6 Easy Steps," Chopra Center, accessed August 25, 2016, http://www.chopra.com/ccl/learn-to-meditate-in-6-easy-steps.

CHAPTER 4

1. Allen Mullen, *An Anatomical Account of the Elephant Accidentally Burnt in Dublin, on Fryday, June 17, in the Year 1681* (London, 1682), 37–41.

2. M. L. Fine et al., "Acanthonus armatus, a Deep-Sea Teleost Fish with a Minute Brain and Large Ears," *Proceedings of the Royal Society B* 230, no. 1259 (1987): 257–265.
3. Michael A. Ward et al., "The Effect of Body Mass Index on Global Brain Volume in Middle-Aged Adults: A Cross Sectional Study," *BioMed Central Neurology* 5 (2005): 23.
4. Majid Fotuhi and Brooke Lubinski, "The Effects of Obesity on Brain Structure and Size," *Practical Neurology* 12, (July/August 2013): 20, http://practicalneurology.com/2013/08/the-effects-of-obesity-on-brain-structure-and-size.
5. T. M. Frayling et al., "A Common Variant in the FTO Gene Is Associated with Body Mass Index and Predisposes to Childhood and Adult Obesity," *Science* 316, no. 5826 (2007): 889–894.
6. April J. Ho, et al., "A Commonly Carried Allele of the Obesity-Related FTO Gene Is Associated with Reduced Brain Volume in the Healthy Elderly," *Proceedings of the National Academy of Sciences of the United States of America* 107.18 (2010): 8404–8409.
7. Ana Navarette et al., "Energetics and the Evolution of Human Brain Size," *Nature* 480, no. 7375 (December 2011): 91–93.
8. Krister Svahn, "Newly-Discovered Human Fat Cell Opens Up New Opportunities for Future Treatment of Obesity," *ScienceDaily*, May 2, 2013, www.sciencedaily.com/releases/2013/05/130502081745.htm.
9. M. P. Jedrychowski et al., "Detection and Quantitation of Circulating Human Irisin by Tandem Mass Spectrometry," *Cell Metabolism* (October 6, 2015) Oct 6; 22(4): 734–40.
10. Marlene Zuk, *Paleofantasy: What Evolution Really Tells Us about Sex, Diet, and How We Live* (New York: W. W. Norton & Company, Inc., 2013), 270.
11. S. Boyd Eaton, "Evolution and Cholesterol," in *A Balanced Omega-6/Omega-3 Fatty Acid Ratio, Cholesterol and Coronary Heart Disease*, eds. A. Simopoulos and F. De Meester (Basel, Switzerland: Karger, 2009), 47.
12. Lorna T. Corr and Richard P. Evershed, et al., "Probing Dietary Change of the Kwäday Dän Ts'inchi Individual, an Ancient Glacier Body from British Columbia: I. Complementary Use of Marine Lipid Biomarker and Carbon Isotope Signatures as Novel Indicators of a Marine Diet," *Journal of Archaeological Science* 35, no. 8 (August 2008): 2102–10.
13. Artemis P. Simopoulos and Leslie G. Cleland, ed., "Omega–6/Omega–3 Essential Fatty Acid Ratio: The Scientific Evidence World," *Review of Nutrition and Dietetics*, ISSN 0084–2230, vol. 92, S. Karger AG Publications (2003): chapter 4009.
14. James Gallagher, "Processed Meats Do Cause Cancer—WHO," *BBC Health* (October 26, 2015): http://www.bbc.com/news/health-34615621.
15. Stephen C. Cunnane, *Survival of the Fattest: The Key to Human Brain Evolution* (Hackensack, NJ: World Scientific Publishing Co., 2005).
16. Mark Bricklin, *The Diabetes Rescue Diet: Conquer Diabetes Naturally While Eating and Drinking What You Love—Even Chocolate and Wine!* (Emmaus, PA: Rodale Books, 2013), 52.

17. United States Department of Agriculture and the United States Department of Health and Human Services, *Dietary Guidelines for Americans* (Washington, DC: United States Government Printing Office, 2010): 25.

18. United States Department of Agriculture, Agricultural Research Service, Nutrient Stat Laboratory, "USDA National Nutrient Database for Standard Reference, Release 16," 2003, accessed October 13, 2016, http://www.ars.usda.gov/main/site_main .htm?modecode=80-40-05-25.

19. Henry J. Thompson and Mark A. Brick, "Perspective: Closing the Dietary Fiber Gap: An Ancient Solution for a 21st Century Problem," *Advances in Nutrition* 7 (2016): 623–6; doi:10.3945/an.115.009696.

20. Zoe Harcombe et al., "Evidence from Randomised Controlled Trials Did Not Support the Introduction of Dietary Fat Guidelines in 1977 and 1983: A Systematic Review and Meta-Analysis," *Open Heart* 2, no. 1 (2015).

21. Ibid.

22. L. M. Nackers et al., "The Association between Rate of Initial Weight Loss and Long-Term Success in Obesity Treatment: Does Slow and Steady Win the Race?" *International Journal of Behavioral Medicine* 17, no. 3 (2010): 161–167.

23. George Eliot, *Middlemarch* (New York: Penguin Classics, 2003), 76.

24. David Wismer, "Gov. Chris Christie: 'I'm Basically the Healthiest Fat Guy You've Ever Seen' (And Other Quotes of the Week)," *Forbes*, February 10, 2013, http://www .forbes.com/sites/davidwismer/2013/02/10/gov-chris-christie-im-basically-the -healthiest-fat-guy-youve-ever-seen-and-other-quotes-of-the-week/#5a3a32032be6.

25. Kirsty Spalding et al., "Dynamics of Fat Cell Turnover in Humans," *Nature* 453 (2008): 783–787.

26. Krushnapriya Sahoo et al., "Childhood Obesity: Causes and Consequences," *Journal of Family Medicine and Primary Care* 4.2 (2015): 187–92.

27. Christopher Kuzawa, "Adipose Tissue in Human Infancy and Childhood: An Evolutionary Perspective," *Yearbook of Physical Anthropology* 41 (1998): 181.

28. Stephen S. Hall, "Our Closest Relative among Model Organisms: Discovering the Obesity Genes," *The Genes We Share*, Howard Hughes Medical Institute, 2008, accessed July 1, 2016, http://webprojects.oit.ncsu.edu/project/bio181de/Black/endo-crine2/endocrine2_reading/d130.html.

29. Rebecca Perl, "How Leptin Rewires the Brain," *The Rockefeller University Scientist*, May 14, 2004, http://www.rockefeller.edu/pubinfo/news_notes/rus_051404_c.php.

30. Robert H. Lustig, *Fat Chance: Beating the Odds Against Sugar, Processed Food, Obesity, and Disease* (New York: Plume, 2013).

31. John A. Matochik et al., "Effect of Leptin Replacement on Brain Structure in Genetically Leptin-Deficient Adults," *Journal of Clinical Endocrinology and Metabolism* 90, no. 5 (2005): 2851–2854.

32. M. K. Serdula et al., "Do Obese Children Become Obese Adults? A Review of the Literature," *Preventative Medicine* 22, no. 2 (1993): 167–177.

33. "Good vs. Bad Cholesterol," *American Heart Association*, updated March 23, 2016, http://www.heart.org/HEARTORG/Conditions/Cholesterol/AboutCholesterol /Good-vs-Bad-Cholesterol_UCM_305561_Article.jsp#.Vi2pHXhuaEl.

34. P. Lindström et al., "The Physiology of Obese-Hyperglycemic Mice [ob/ob mice]," *The Scientific World Journal* 7 (2007): 666–685.
35. Ernest Becker, *The Denial of Death* (New York: Free Press, 1973), 12.
36. Daniel Steinberg, *The Cholesterol Wars: The Skeptics vs. the Preponderance of Evidence* (Amsterdam: Academic Press, 2007), 17.
37. Daniel Steinberg, "In Celebration of the 100th Anniversary of the Lipid Hypothesis of Atherosclerosis," *Journal of Lipid Research* 54.11 (2013): 2946–2949.
38. Truswell A. Stewart, "De Langen in Dutch East Indies 1916–1922," *Cholesterol and Beyond: The Research on Diet and Coronary Heart Disease 1900–2000* (New York: Springer, 2010) 39.
39. J. Groen et al., "Influence of Nutrition, Individual, and Some Other Factors, Including Various Forms of Stress, on Serum Cholesterol; Experiment of Nine Months' Duration in 60 Normal Human Volunteers," *Voeding* 13 (1952): 556–87.
40. Ancel Keys, "Effects of Diet on Blood Lipids in Man: Particularly Cholesterol and Lipoproteins," *Clinical Chemistry* 1, no. 1 (1955): 34–52.
41. Daniel Steinberg, "In Celebration of the 100th Anniversary of the Lipid Hypothesis of Atherosclerosis," *The Journal of Lipid Research* 54, no. 11 (2013): 2946–2949.
42. M. F. Muldoon, "Acute Cholesterol Responses to Mental Stress and Change in Posture," *Archives of Internal Medicine* 152, no. 4 (1992): 775–780.
43. P. Mani and A. Rohatgi, "Niacin Therapy, HDL Cholesterol, and Cardiovascular Disease: Is the HDL Hypothesis Defunct?" *Current Atherosclerosis Reports* 17, no. 8 (2015): 43.
44. Michael O'Riordan, "New Cholesterol Guidelines Abandon LDL Targets," *Medscape*, November 12, 2013, http://www.medscape.com/viewarticle/814152.
45. American College of Cardiology/American Heart Association Task Force on Practice Guidelines, "2013 ACC/AHA Guideline on the Treatment of Blood Cholesterol to Reduce Atherosclerotic Cardiovascular Risk in Adults," American College of Cardiology/American Heart Association 129 (2014): S1-S45, https://doi.org/10.1161/01 .cir.0000437738.63853.7a circulation.
46. Francisco Lopez-Jimenez, M.D., "Eggs: Are They Good or Bad for My Cholesterol," Mayo Clinic, accessed August 1, 2016, http://www.mayoclinic.org/diseases-conditions /high-blood-cholesterol/expert-answers/cholesterol/faq-20058468.
47. Ibid.
48. Ancel Keys, "Letter to the Editor: Normal Plasma Cholesterol in a Man Who Eats 25 Eggs a Day" *New England Journal of Medicine* 325 (August 22, 1991): 584. http:// www.nejm.org/doi/full/10.1056/NEJM199108223250813#t=article.
49. L. J. Whalley et al., "Plasma Vitamin C, Cholesterol and Homocysteine Are Associated with Gray Matter Volume Determined by MRI in Non-Demented Old People," *Neuroscience Letters* 341, no. 3 (2003): 173–176.
50. Joseph Friedman et al., "Brain Imaging Changes Associated with Risk Factors for Cardiovascular and Cerebrovascular Disease in Asymptomatic Patients," *Journal of the American College of Cardiovascular Imaging* 7, no. 10 (2014): 1039–1053.
51. Mireille Guiliano, *French Women Don't Get Fat* (New York: Doubleday, 2004).

52. D. Corella et al., "APOA2, Dietary Fat, and Body Mass Index: Replication of a Gene-Diet Interaction in 3 Independent Populations," *Archives of Internal Medicine* 169, no. 20 (2009): 1897–1906.

53. Moyra Mortby et al., "High 'Normal' Blood Glucose Is Associated with Decreased Brain Volume and Cognitive Performance in the 60s: The PATH through Life Study," *PLoS ONE* 8, no. 9 (2013): e73697.

54. T. Kazumi et al., "Effects of Dietary Fructose or Glucose on Triglyceride Production and Lipogenic Enzyme Activities in the Liver of Wistar Fatty Rats, an Animal Model of NIDDM," *Endocrinology Journal* 44, no. 2 (1997): 239–245.

55. Arline Kaplan, "Statins, Cholesterol Depletion—and Mood Disorders: What's the Link," *Psychiatric Times*, November 30, 2010, http://www.psychiatrictimes.com/mood-disorders/statins-cholesterol-depletion—and-mood-disorders-what's-link.

56. Beatrice A. Golomb et al., "Statin Effects on Aggression: Results from the UCSD Statin Study, a Randomized Control Trial," *PLOS ONE*, July 1, 2015, http://journals.plos.org/plosone/article?id=10.1371/journal.pone.0124451.

57. John Naish, "Why Your Pills May Be Making You Angry: As Statins Are Linked to Aggression in Women, the Mood-Altering Side-Effects of Everyday Medicines," *Daily Mail*, July 13, 2015, http://www.dailymail.co.uk/health/article-3159774/Why-pills-making-angry-statins-linked-aggression-women-mood-altering-effects-every-day-medicines.html.

58. Aristotle quoted in *Quote Junkie: Greek and Roman Edition* (Dayton, OH: Hagopian Institute, 2008), 7.

CHAPTER 5

1. V. M. Sheth and A. G. Pandya, "Melasma: A Comprehensive Update: Part I," *Journal of the American Academy of Dermatology* 65, no. 4 (2011): 689–697.

2. Charles Darwin, *The Descent of Man and Selection in Relation to Sex*, 2nd ed. (London, 1874), 604.

3. C. G. Seligman, *Races of Africa* (London: Thornton Butterworth Ltd., 1930), 96.

4. Samuel Stanhope Smith, *An Essay on the Causes of the Variety of Complexion and Figure in the Human Species*, ed. Winthrop D. Jordan (New York: Harvard University Press, 1965).

5. George Sebastian Rousseau, "Le Cat and the Physiology of Negroes," *Enlightenment Crossings: Pre- and Post-modern Discourses* (Manchester: UK, Manchester University Press, 1991) 37.

6. K. F. Heusinger, "Untersuchungen ueber die Anomalie der Kohlenund Pigmentbildung in dem menschlichen Kôrper," *System der Histologie* (Germany, 1823).

7. Martine F. Luxwolda et al., "Traditionally Living Populations in East Africa Have a Mean Serum 25-Hydroxyvitamin D Concentration of 115 nmol/l," *British Journal of Nutrition* 108, no. 9 (2012): 1557–1561.

8. Darwin, *Descent of Man*, 192.

9. Jöns Jacob Berzelius, quoted in *The Study of Chemical Composition*, Ida Freund (Cambridge: Cambridge University Press, 1904), 31.

10. Jerry Bergman, "ATP: The Perfect Energy Currency," *Creation Research Society Quarterly* 36, no. 1 (1999): 3.

11. Philip Larkin, *The Less Deceived* (Hessle, England: The Marvell Press, 1955), "Skin."

12. Franscesco Visioli et al., "Dietary Intake of Fish vs. Formulations Leads to Higher Plasma Concentrations of n-3 Fatty Acids," *Lipids* 38, no. 4 (2003): 415–418.

13. W. S. Harris et al., "Comparison of Effects of Fish and Fish-Oil Capsules on the n-3 Fatty Acid Content of Blood Cells and Plasma Phospholipids," *American Journal of Clinical Nutrition* 86, no. 6 (2007): 1621–1625.

14. A. Lucas et al., "Breast Milk and Subsequent Intelligence Quotient in Children Born Preterm" *Lancet* 339, no. 8788 (1992): 261–264.

15. M. P. Judge et al., "Maternal Consumption of a Docosahexaenoic Acid-Containing Functional Food During Pregnancy: Benefit for Infant Performance on Problem-Solving, but Not on Recognition Memory Tasks at Age 9 Months," *American Journal of Clinical Nutrition* 85, no. 6 (2007): 1572–1577.

16. United States Department of Agriculture and the United States Department of Health and Human Services, *Dietary Guidelines for Americans* (Washington, DC: United States Government Printing Office, 2010).

17. Harvard Health Publications, "Why Not Flaxseed Oil?" *The Family Health Guide*, updated November 2006, http://www.health.harvard.edu/staying-healthy/why-not-flaxseed-oil.

18. S. C. Cottin et al., "The Differential Effects of EPA and DHA on Cardiovascular Risk Factors," *Proceedings of the Nutrition Society* 70, no. 2 (2011): 215–231.

19. W. S. An et al., "Omega-3 Fatty Acid Supplementation Increases 1,25-Dihydroxyvitamin D and Fetuin-A Levels in Dialysis Patients," *Nutrition Research* 32, no. 7 (2012): 495–502.

20. Josefina López, *Unconquered Spirits: A Historical Play* (Woodstock, IL: Dramatic Publishing, 1997), 63.

21. Jose Andres Puerta, Royal Culinary Academy of Arts Facebook page, accessed July 25, 2016, https://www.facebook.com/RACAJordan/posts/10153090358616850.

22. M. K. Bogh et al., "Vitamin D Production Depends on Ultraviolet-B Dose but Not on Dose Rate: A Randomized Controlled Trial," *Experimental Dermatology* 20, no. 1 (2011): 14–18.

23. J. A. Newton-Bishop et al., "Serum 25-Hydroxyvitamin D3 Levels Are Associated with Breslow Thickness at Presentation and Survival from Melanoma," *Journal of Clinical Oncology* 27, no. 32 (2009): 5439–5444.

CHAPTER 6

1. Jennifer Donnelly, *Revolution* (New York: Ember, 2011), 5.

2. Danielle Reed et al, "Diverse Tastes: Genetics of sweet and bitter perception," *Physiology & Behavior* 88, no. 3 (2006): 215–226.

3. Qais Al-Awqati, "Evidence-Based Politics of Salt and Blood Pressure," *Kidney International* 69, no. 10 (2006): 1707–1708.

4. P. A. Breslin et al., "Suppression of Bitterness by Sodium: Variation among Bitter Taste Stimuli," *Chemical Senses* 20 (1995): 609–623.

5. Graham Macgregor et al. "Commentary: Salt, Blood Pressure and Health," *International Journal of Epidemiology* 31, no. 2 (2002): 320–327.

6. N. J. Aburto et al., "Effect of Lower Sodium Intake on Health: Systematic Review and Meta-Analyses," *British Medical Journal* 346 (2013): f1326.

7. G. K. Beauchamp and K. Engelman, "High Salt Intake. Sensory and Behavioral Factors," *Hypertension* 17, no. 1 Suppl. (1991): 1176–1181; M. J. Brion et al., "Sodium Intake in Infancy and Blood Pressure at 7 Years: Findings from the Avon Longitudinal Study of Parents and Children," *European Journal of Clinical Nutrition* 62, no. 10 (2008): 1162–69.

8. Graham MacGregor, "Salt: Neptune's Poisoned Chalice," lecture at Barts and the London School of Medicine and Dentistry, accessed March 1, 2016, http://www.smd .qmul.ac.uk/events/publichealthprimarycare/macgregor/43919.html.

9. Ibid.

10. Ibid.

11. E. Poch et al., "Molecular Basis of Salt Sensitivity in Human Hypertension. Evaluation of Renin-Angiotensin-Aldosterone System Gene Polymorphisms," *Hypertension* 38, no. 5 (2001): 1204–1209.

12. Serge Daget, An Englishman Tastes the Sweat of an African (1725), reproduced in M. J. Brown, "Hypertension and Ethnic Group," *British Medical Journal* 332, no. 7545 (date): 833.

13. Flávio D. Fuchs, "Why Do Black Americans Have Higher Prevalence of Hypertension? An Enigma Still Unsolved," *Hypertension* 57 (2011): 379–380.

14. United States Department of Agriculture, "Sodium (Salt) Content of Common Foods," accessed March 1, 2016, http://www.jdabrams.com/documents/wellness/ USDA-Sodium-Content.pdf.

15. H. Basciano et al., "Fructose, Insulin Resistance, and Metabolic Dyslipidemia," *Nutrition & Metabolism* 2, no. 1 (2005); A. Astrup and N. Finer, "Redefining Type 2 Diabetes: 'Diabesity' or 'Obesity Dependent Diabetes Mellitus'?" *Obesity Review* 1, no. 2 (2000): 57–59.

16. "Evolutionary Biology: Sugar Sweetens Cell Cooperation," *Nature* 476, no. 7360 (2011): 254.

17. Maude W. Baldwin et al., "Evolution of Sweet Taste Perception in Hummingbirds by Transformation of the Ancestral Umami Receptor," *Science* 345, no. 6199 (2014): 929–933.

18. Justin Rhodes, "Research Shows Fructose Increases Body Fat and Decreases Physical Activity," Beckman Institute NeuroTech Group, June 1, 2015, http://beckman.illinois. edu/news/2015/06/rhodes-fructose.

19. Nicole M. Avena et al., "Sugar and Fat Bingeing Have Notable Differences in Addictive-Like Behavior," *The Journal of Nutrition* 139, no. 3 (2009): 623–628.

20. "US and Global Obesity Levels: The Fat Chart," ProCon.org, accessed March 1, 2016, http://obesity.procon.org/view.resource.php?resourceID=004371#8.

21. Alison Hughes, "Sweet Tooth? Come to Ireland!" Vagabond Tours, August 27, 2015, https://vagabondtoursofireland.com/sweet-tooth-come-to-ireland/.

22. Anthony Saliba, "Sweet Taste Preference and Personality Traits Using a White Wine," *Food Quality and Preference* 20, no. 8 (2009): 572–575.

23. Karen Eny et al., "Genetic Variant in the Glucose Transporter Type 2 Is Associated with Higher Intakes of Sugars in Two Distinct Populations," *Physiological Genomics* 33, no. 3 (2008): 355–360.

24. Health Canada, *Nutrient Value of Some Common Foods* (Ottawa, Ontario: Health Canada, 2008), 21, 47–49, 52.

25. "Starchy Diet, Extra Genes: Humans Just Keep on Evolving," Stanford at The Tech: Understanding Genetics, 2013, accessed March 1, 2016, http://genetics.thetech.org /original_news/news62.

26. Eric Axelsson et al., "The Genomic Signature of Dog Domestication Reveals Adaptation to a Starch-Rich Diet," *Nature* 495, no. 7441 (2013): 360–364.

27. "GI-Glycaemia Index," NZ Nutrition Foundation, 2009, accessed July 1, 2016, http:// www.nutritionfoundation.org.nz/nutrition-facts/nutrition-a-z/gi-and-gl.

28. G. Riccardi, "Glycemic Index of Local Foods and Diets: The Mediterranean Experience," *Nutrition Review* 61, no. 5 (2003): S56–60.

29. "In Defence of Potatoes," *The Sydney Morning Herald*, August 9, 2011, http:// www.smh.com.au/lifestyle/diet-and-fitness/chew-on-this/in-defence-of-potatoes -20110808-1iirt.html.

30. Janette Brand-Miller et al., "Rice: A High or Low Glycemic Index Food?" *The American Journal of Clinical Nutrition* 56, no. 6 (1992): 1034–1036.

31. Bruna Letícia Pereira and Magali Leonel, "Resistant Starch in Cassava Products," *Food Science and Technology (Campinas)* 34, no. 2 (June 20, 2014): 298–302.

32. Glen Fernandes et al., "Glycemic Index of Potatoes Commonly Consumed in North America," *Journal of the American Dietetic Association* 105, no. 4 (2005): 557–562.

33. "Glycemic Index and Glycemic Load for 100+ Foods: Measuring Carbohydrate Effects Can Help Glucose Management," Harvard Health Publications (February 2015): http://www.health.harvard.edu/diseases-and-conditions/glycemic _index_and_glycemic_load_for_100_foods.

34. M. C. Cornelis et al., "TCF7L2, Dietary Carbohydrate, and Risk of Type 2 Diabetes in US Women," *American Journal of Clinical Nutrition* 89, no. 4 (2009): 1256–1262.

35. A. L. Mandel and P. A. Breslin, "High Endogenous Salivary Amylase Activity Is Associated with Improved Glycemic Homeostasis Following Starch Ingestion in Adults," *Journal of Nutrition* 142, no. 5 (2012): 853–858.

36. Caleb Kelly and Venu Gangur, "Sex Disparity in Food Allergy: Evidence from the PubMed Database," *Journal of Allergy* (2009): https://www.hindawi.com/journals /ja/2009/159845/.

37. Heenashree Khandelwal, *Soulmates, By Chance* (Assam, India: Mahaveer Publications, 2013).

38. Louis Duhring, "Dermatitis Herpetiformis," *Journal of the American Medical Association* 3, no. 9 (1884): 225–229.

39. Diana Gitig, "When, and Why, Did Everyone Stop Eating Gluten?" *Scientific American Blog*, May 10, 2011, http://blogs.scientificamerican.com/guest-blog /when-and-why-did-everyone-stop-eating-gluten.

40. Marianna Karamanou and G. Androutsos, "Aretaeus of Cappadocia and the First Clinical Description of Asthma," *American Journal of Respiratory and Critical Care Medicine* 184, no. 12 (2011): 1420–1421; F. Henschen, "On the Term Diabetes in the Works of Aretaeus and Galen," Medical History 13, no. 2 (1969): 190–192.

41. W. K. Dicke, *Coeliac Diseas. Investigation of the Harmful Effects of Certain Types of Cereal on Patients with Coeliac Disease (Thesis)* (The Netherlands: University of Utrecht, 1950): 23–27.

42. Francis Adams, *The Extant Works of Aretaeus the Cappadocian* (London: Sydenham Society, 1856), 350.

43. Gitig, "When, and Why, Did Everyone Stop Eating Gluten?"

44. Anna Sapone et al., "Divergence of gut permeability and mucosal immune gene expression in two gluten-associated conditions: celiac disease and gluten sensitivity," *BMC Medicine* 9, no. 23 (2011).

45. Novak Djokovic, *Serve to Win: The 14-Day Gluten-Free Plan for Physical and Mental Excellence* (New York: Zinc Ink, 2013), xxv.

46. "Sources of Gluten," Celiac Disease Foundation, accessed September 15, 2016, https:// celiac.org/live-gluten-free/glutenfreediet/sources-of-gluten/.

47. C. A. Adebamowo et al., "Milk Consumption and Acne in Adolescent Girls," *Dermatology Online Journal* 12, no 4 (2006): 1.

48. Andrew Curry, "Archaeology: The Milk Revolution," *Nature* 500, no. 7460 (2013): 20–22.

49. Jared Diamond, "The Worst Mistake in the History of the Human Race," *Discover*, May 1, 1999, http://discovermagazine.com/1987/may/02-the-worst-mistake-in-the -history-of-the-human-race.

50. Ibid.

51. B. G. Maegraith et al., "Suppression of Malaria (P. berghei) by Milk," *British Medical Journal* 2, no. 4799 (1952): 1382–1384.

52. Maryam Alizadeh and A. Sadr-Nabavi, "Evaluation of a Genetic Test for Diagnose of Primary Hypolactasia in Northeast of Iran (Khorasan)," *Iranian Journal of Basic Medical Sciences* 15, no. 6 (2012): 1127–1130.

53. Elie Roe, "Is Lactose Intolerance on the Rise?" *Science in Our World: Certainty and Controversy*, September 19, 2013, http://www.personal.psu.edu/afr3/blogs /siowfa13/2013/09/is-lactose-intolerance-on-the-rise.html.

54. "Scientific Opinion on Lactose Thresholds in Lactose Intolerance and Galactosaemia," *European Food Safety Authority Journal* 8, no. 9 (2010), 1777.

55. Capcom, *Ace Attorney*, Giant Bomb, accessed July 25, 2016, http://www.giantbomb. com/godot/3005-2706/.

56. Dietitians of Canada, "Food Sources of Lactose," dieticians.ca, http://www.dietitians .ca/Your-Health/Nutrition-A-Z/Lactose/Food-Sources-of-Lactose.aspx.

57. Amie J. Dirks-Naylor, "The Benefits of Coffee on Skeletal Muscle," *Life Sciences* 143 (2015): 182–186.

58. Nina Luttinger and Gregory Dicum, *The Coffee Book: Anatomy of an Industry from Crop to the Last Drop* (New York: The New Press, 2006): 2–3.

59. Roger Clavill, *Happiness Improved, Or, An Infallible Way to Get Riches, Encrease Plenty, and Promote Pleasure* (London, Roger Clavil, 1697) chapter VI, 95.

60. E. J. Welsh et al., "Caffeine for Asthma," *Cochrane Database of Systematic Reviews* no. 1 (2010).

61. A. L. Klatsky et al., "Coffee, Tea, and Mortality," *Annals of Epidemiology* 3, no. 4 (1993): 375–381.

62. Michel Lucas et al., "Coffee, Caffeine, and Risk of Completed Suicide: Results from three Prospective Cohorts of American Adults," *The World Journal of Biological Psychiatry* 15, no. 5 (2014): 382.

63. Sheena Derry et al., "Single Dose Oral Ibuprofen Plus Caffeine for Acute Postoperative Pain in Adults," *The Cochrane Database of Systematic Reviews* no. 7 (2015).

64. Joseph Stromberg, "This Is How Your Brain Becomes Addicted to Caffeine" Smithsonian.com, August 9, 2013, http://www.smithsonianmag.com/science-nature/this-is-how-your-brain-becomes-addicted-to-caffeine-26861037/?no-ist.

65. Pertti Happonen et al., "Coffee Drinking Is Dose-Dependently Related to the Risk of Acute Coronary Events in Middle-Aged Men," *The Journal of Nutrition* 134, no. 9 (2004): http://jn.nutrition.org/content/134/9/2381.full.

66. Ahmed El-Sohemy et al., "Coffee, CYP1A2 Genotype, and Risk of Myocardial Infarction," *The Journal of the American Medical Association* 295, no. 10 (March 8, 2006): 1135–1141.

67. Ivana Hečimović et al., "Comparative Study of Polyphenols and Caffeine in Different Coffee Varieties Affected by the Degree of Roasting," *Food Chemistry* 129, no. 3 (2011): 991–1000.

68. H. N. Wanyika et al., "Determination of Caffeine Content of Tea and Instant Coffee Brands Found in the Kenyan Market," *African Journal of Food Science* 4, no. 6 (2010): 353–358.

69. Rachel R. McCusker et al., "Caffeine Content of Decaffeinated Coffee," *Journal of Analytical Toxicology* 30, no. 8 (October 2006): 611–613; Ivana Hečimović et al., "Comparative Study of Polyphenols and Caffeine in Different Coffee Varieties Affected by the Degree of Roasting," *Food Chemistry* 129, no. 3 (December 2011): 991–1000; Ben Desbrow et al., "An Examination of Consumer Exposure to Caffeine from Retail Coffee Outlets," *Food and Chemical Toxicology* 45, no. 9 (September 2007): 1588–1592.

70. Aleksandr Solzhenitsyn, H. T. Willetts, trans., *August 1914: The Red Wheel* (New York, Farrar, Straus and Giroux, 2000) ch. 42.

71. D. I. Harvie, Limeys: *The True Story of One Man's War Against Ignorance, the Establishment and the Deadly Scurvy* (Stroud, UK: The History Press, 2002), 12.

72. "The Observations of Sir Richard Hawkins, Knight, in His Voyage into the South Sea, Annodomini, 1593," *Nutrition Reviews* 44, no. 11 (1986): 370–371.

73. C. P. Stewart and D. Gutrie, eds., *Lind's Treatise on Scurvy: A Bicentary Volume* (Edinburgh: Edinburgh University Press, 1953), 440.

74. Ibid.

75. Ganesh N. Dakhale et al., "Supplementation of Vitamin C Reduces Blood Glucose and Improves Glycosylated Hemoglobin in Type 2 Diabetes Mellitus: A Randomized, Double-Blind Study," *Advances in Pharmacological Sciences* (2011): https://www.hindawi.com/journals/aps/2011/195271/.

76. "Drugs and Supplements, Vitamin C (Ascorbic Acid): Dosing," Mayo Clinic, last updated November 1, 2013, http://www.mayoclinic.org/drugs-supplements /vitamin-c/dosing/hrb-20060322.

77. A. Horska et al., "Vitamin C Levels in Blood Are Influenced by Polymorphisms in Glutathione S-Transferases," *European Journal of Nutrition* 50, no. 6 (2011): 437–446.

78. Dietitians of Canada, "Food Sources of Vitamin C," dietitians.ca, February 25, 2014, http://www.dietitians.ca/Your-Health/Nutrition-A-Z/Vitamins/Food-Sources-of -Vitamin-C.aspx.

79. "Micronutrient Deficiencies: Vitamin A Deficiency," World Health Organization, accessed March 1, 2016, http://www.who.int/nutrition/topics/vad/en/.

80. "Vitamin A: Fact Sheet for Health Professionals," National Institutes of Health Office of Dietary Supplements, updated February 11, 2016, https://ods.od.nih.gov /factsheets/VitaminA-HealthProfessional/.

81. Daily Iron, "Iron content of Pumpkin Pie Spice," DailyIron.net, accessed August 25, 2016, http://www.dailyiron.net/pumpkin-pie-spice/.

82. Geoffrey Chaucer, *The Canterbury Tales: A Reader-Friendly Version Put into Modern Spelling by Michael Murphy*," (New York: Brooklyn College) 22, line 500: http://academic.brooklyn.cuny.edu/webcore/murphy/canterbury/2genpro.pdf, accessed Jan 9, 2017.

83. A. L. Schade and L. Caroline, "Raw Hen Egg White and the Role of Iron in Growth Inhibition of Shigella Dysenteriae, Staphylococcus Aureus, Escherichia Coli and Saccharomyces Cerevisiae," *Science* 100, no. 2584 (1944): 14–15.

84. E. D. Weinberg, "Nutritional Immunity. Host's Attempt to Withhold Iron from Microbial Invaders," *Journal of the American Medical Association* 231, no. 1 (1975): 39–41.

85. George Cartwright et al., "The Anaemia of Chronic Disorders," *British Journal of Haematology* 21, no. 2 (1971): 147–152, doi: 10.1111/j.1365-2141.1971.tb03424.x.

86. Lewis Carroll, *Alice's Adventures in Wonderland & Through the Looking-Glass* (New York: Bantam Classics, 1984), 135.

87. S. Sazawal et al., "Effects of Routine Prophylactic Supplementation with Iron and Folic Acid on Admission to Hospital and Mortality in Preschool Children in a High Malaria Transmission Setting: Community-Based, Randomized, Placebo-Controlled Trial," *Lancet* 367, no. 9505 (2006): 133–143.

88. Bradley Wertheim, "The Iron in Our Blood that Keeps and Kills Us," *The Atlantic*, January 10, 2013, http://www.theatlantic.com/health/archive/2013/01/the-iron-in -our-blood-that-keeps-and-kills-us/266936/.

89. K. J. Allen et al., "Iron-Overload-Related Disease in HFE Hereditary Hemochromatosis," *New England Journal of Medicine* 358 (2008): 221–30; I. Pichler et al., "Identification of a Common Variant in the TFR2 Gene Implicated in the Physiolog-

ical Regulation of Serum Iron Levels," *Human Molecular Genetics* 15, no. 6 (2011): 1232–40.

90. United States Department of Agriculture, "Dietary Reference Intakes for Vitamin A, Vitamin K, Arsenic, Boron, Chromium, Copper, Iodine, Iron, Manganese, Molybdenum, Nickel, Silicon, Vanadium, and Zinc," United States Department of Agriculture, accessed July 1, 2016, https://fnic.nal.usda.gov/food-composition /vitamins-and-minerals.

91. Health Canada, *Nutrient Value of Some Common Foods* (Ottawa, Ontario: Health Canada, 2008), 21, 47–49, 52

CONCLUSION

1. Michael P. Garogalo et al., "Hands On: Fingers and Hands and Skin Touch, Feeling Manipulating, Sensing Eye-Hand Coordination, Tool Using, Somaesthetics Identity and Actions, Self and Praxis, Language and Touch," updated March 15, 2013, http:// www.egreenway.com/reason/touch.htm.

2. Linda Rosa et al., "A Close Look at Therapeutic Touch," *Journal of the American Medical Association*, 279, no. 13 (1998): 1005–1010.

3. Saint Augustine, Quotes.net, accessed August 1, 2016, http://www.quotes.net /authors/Saint Augustine.

4. Nelson Mandela, *Long Walk to Freedom: Autobiography of Nelson Mandela* (New York: Back Bay Books, 1995), 391.

5. François Rabelais, *Five Books of the Lives, Heroic Deeds and Sayings of Gargantua and His Son Pantagruel, Volume III* (London: A. H. Bullen, 1904), 14.

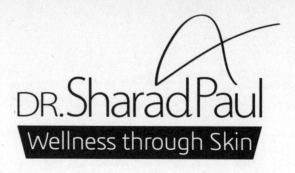

DR. Sharad Paul
Wellness through Skin

Would you like to know if you are better suited to endurance or power sports? Or do you only want to know if you can continue to drink several cups of coffee a day and not increase your risk of heart disease?

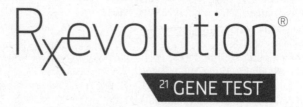

R$_x$evolution ®
²¹ GENE TEST

My team will analyze your genetic code and determine how your genes can influence your stress levels, nutrient or mineral metabolism, and sports preferences. Most importantly, you can learn to "eat for your gene type." Upon ordering (kits cost $299) a test-kit will be mailed to you with details of your closest lab to send a saliva sample to, and you will (in about 4 weeks) receive a personalized, comprehensive report that can help you take charge of your own health.

TEST YOUR GENES NOW AT:
www.geneticsofhealth.com

Dr. Sharad Paul's R$_x$EVOLUTION® 21-Gene Testing Program is meant to provide general health advice, and not intended as treatment for medical conditions. Therefore, US FDA approval has not been sought or obtained. If you have questions, please contact us.